Mal de Debarquement Syndrome

A Comprehensive Patient Guide

Mal de Debarquement Syndrome: A Comprehensive Patient Guide

Mark Knoblauch PhD

Kiremma Press
Houston, TX

© 2019 by Mark Knoblauch

Printed in the United States of America

<u>Disclaimer</u>: The information provided within this book is for general informational purposes only. While the author tries to keep the information up-to-date and correct, there are no representations or warranties, express or implied, about the completeness, accuracy, reliability, suitability or availability with respect to the information contained in this book for any purpose. Any use of this information is at your own risk. Furthermore, the methods described within this book are the author's personal thoughts and opinions. As such, they are not intended to be a definitive set of instructions for you to follow precisely. You may discover there are other methods and materials to accomplish the same end result.

www.authorMK.com

ISBN: 978-1-7333210-1-3

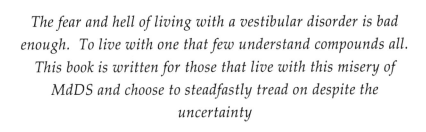

The fear and hell of living with a vestibular disorder is bad enough. To live with one that few understand compounds all. This book is written for those that live with this misery of MdDS and choose to steadfastly tread on despite the uncertainty

Table of Contents

Introduction

Until someone has had the unfortunate experience of chronic dizziness or instability, it's hard to imagine the intrusion and inconvenience that often accompanies such frustrating symptoms. What used to be a quick trip to the store in one's healthier days might now be considered an impossible task, or at least one that requires significant preparation and a likely list of Plans B, C, and D in the event that something goes wrong along the way. For many individuals, even chores around the house can become dreaded tasks after the onset of a disorder that affects their equilibrium. The handicap of the disorder can often be tied in with repeated cancellations, avoidance of public areas, and a general withdrawal from society, all of which can be compounded by a degree of misunderstanding or even lack of sympathy from friends and family due to the fact that many dizziness-based disorders lack outward signs that others can see. This often leaves the affected individual trapped in a world that only they can experience, with their disorder leaving them to deal with a variety of good and bad days and perhaps even a few symptom-free days likely mixed in. Others may experience an ongoing degree of misery at all hours. The unpredictability can often be the most frustrating part. This, in a nutshell, is life with a chronic vestibular disorder.

Depending on the patient's affliction, there may be a wealth of information available for outlining the disease – even if there is not a clear path to recovery. For example, research into vestibular-based conditions such as the relatively common benign paroxysmal positional vertigo (BPPV) has led to a simple maneuver-based treatment that works for the vast majority of patients. Similarly, acoustic neuroma research has now developed a 'watch and wait' treatment plan for patients that involves monitoring the tumor over time, even though there is clear evidence of a tumor existing within their skull. Other related conditions may have recognizable symptoms but no consistently effective treatment. Vestibular migraine, Ménière's disease, and persistent postural-perceptual dizziness (PPPD) are a few well-known dizziness- or instability-based conditions that present somewhat similar across patients but do not have a clearly-recognized treatment plan. In recent years, Mal de Debarquement Syndrome (MdDS) has joined this list of instability-related conditions that present with a particular set of symptoms but does not yet have a clearly outlined treatment plan. Whereas MdDS is not as common as many other instability-based disorders, those affected by MdDS are often left confused as to the cause, effects, and cascade of events that occur after diagnosis with MdDS. It is those patients for whom this book is written.

As someone who has been diagnosed with multiple vestibular disorders, I know the frustration and even anger that can accompany a medical condition that few know about. I was diagnosed with BPPV almost 20 years ago, and while I've been lucky enough to receive successful treatment of that condition I still deal with symptoms associated with ongoing tinnitus and Ménière's disease as well as a few factors that suggest vestibular migraine. Because of my experience with these conditions, I know full well the annoyance that new patients often have specific to finding a quality source of medical information that is based on facts rather than anecdotes or personal experiences. That frustration, coupled with my research and writing background drove me to write my own set of patient-based medical books in which I compile the latest research on vestibular and dizziness-based disorders and work to condense that research down into a format that can be understood by any patient. What you won't find in my books are personal opinions or any upselling of a product or website membership. My intent is to inform you the patient and arm you with solid information that can help you have an educated discussion with your medical provider.

Given the positive feedback I have received from readers of my previous books, I have elected to continue on with my writing and tackle the condition of MdDS. Even though I have not been 'officially' diagnosed with MdDS, it is clear to others around me that I am more susceptible to a temporary (2+ hours) degree of an increased sensation of motion and rocking after boat rides. Perhaps this is due to a deficiency within my own affected vestibular system, or it may just be a slight malfunction left over from something that I was born with. Either way, my own experience with the annoying sensation of false movement after getting off of a boat has allowed me to understand a small portion of what MdDS patients go through. In turn, my goal in writing this book is to provide solid information and maybe even a bit of psychological relief for those who suffer from MdDS.

To accomplish my goal, this book is broken down into distinct chapters that outline relevant aspects of MdDS. Starting in Chapter 1, we'll take an in-depth look at the systems used by our body to establish our balance and equilibrium, with particular emphasis focused on the vestibular system of the inner ear. Although MdDS's true cause has not been revealed, there is reasonable suspicion that it may be in part linked to feedback received by the balance and movement-sensing structures of the inner ear. Therefore, we'll take a look at how the inner ear's structures detect and transmit signals associated with motion, and we'll also outline how our vision and other sensory systems play a role in our ability to maintain balance.

After looking at our balance systems, we'll next detail out the symptoms of dizziness and seasickness, as both are somewhat related to what sufferers of MdDS experience. With that background information in hand, we'll then explore MdDS as a medical condition. Chapter 3 will outline demographics such as the age and gender of those most affected by MdDS, describe the most common symptoms, and list the suspected causes for MdDS. We'll then look at the current recommended diagnostic criteria used in differentiating MdDS from other dizziness-based conditions, followed by proposed treatments to help improve the effects of MdDS. Lastly, we'll look at how quality of life is affected by MdDS and also outline various other medical conditions that have effects similar to MdDS.

Hopefully, upon reaching the end of this book you will have learned valuable information that not only allows you to understand MdDS better but also empowers you to make positive and helpful decisions specific to your own care. Unfortunately, MdDS does not have the research history that many other equilibrium disorders have; consequently, the degree of what we know specific to treatments, diagnosis, or causes of MdDS does not reach a level shared by conditions such as BPPV or Ménière's disease. Still, as you will read, it is encouraging to know that researchers are actively working to understand how the various balance-detections systems operate as well as how the neural pathways used by the brain process this information.

Certainly, with continued research will come more answers that lead to improved treatments and – hopefully – a cure. Keeping this in mind, much of what we know about MdDS is theoretical or in some cases based on results that occurred in only a few patients. Still, any available information specific to MdDS helps set the groundwork for future, more directed work. Until then, patients must be sure to stay in constant communication with their healthcare provider, informing them of triggers, improvements, or aspects (e.g. diet changes) that affect their MdDS. In the end, we are all working toward the same goal – relief – which takes a proactive patient to inform others about what works and doesn't work. My intent is that this book serves to bring you some explanations, answers, and perhaps encouragement that dealing with MdDS is possible, and that there is hope for improvement on the horizon. Sometimes, just knowing that there are people out there working for you can be a beneficial light in the very dark world of vestibular disorders.

With that being said, let's get started on your journey to learning more about the miserable condition of MdDS.

Chapter 1: Perception of Motion

Truth be told, researchers just don't yet know what causes MdDS. The suspected culprit has been narrowed down a bit to what researchers believe are areas of the body that regulate balance or equilibrium, but currently there is not a particular structure that has been identified as being responsible for triggering the effects of MdDS. There are suspicions that MdDS is involved with an intricate mix of neural pathways, reflexes, vestibular input, and/or specific areas of the brain, but further research is needed to outline just which of these is most involved, or if perhaps they all contribute in some way. We could easily spend several chapters outlining complex details about each of the suspected systems that contribute to MdDS, but that would create an exhausting amount of issues to discuss such as muscle spindles, complex nerve pathways, and even an overview of our vision system that would likely lead to this book resembling more of an academic textbook than a patient guide. Instead, we'll focus this chapter predominantly on just a couple of systems that influence our ability to maintain equilibrium, with most emphasis geared towards the vestibular system given that MdDS has been said to likely originate from within the vestibular system[1]. While there may be an interplay of other systems that influence the symptoms associated with MdDS, the vestibular system provides a good starting point as it is intimately involved in our ability to maintain equilibrium. Therefore, we'll use this chapter to outline the vestibular system as well as a couple of other systems that our body relies on to maintain balance.

The vestibular system

The inner ear, located deep within our temporal bone, is responsible for two major roles in our body. One of these roles is specific to that portion of the inner ear dedicated to our sense of hearing, particularly in detecting and converting sound waves to neural impulses. The second role of the inner ear is to detect movement of the head and relay that information to the brain. This dual role that the inner ear plays makes it not only a highly important part of our anatomy but also one that can cause significant disability when it is not functioning correctly. In fact, because of its high level of involvement in detecting sound and motion, the inner ear has been called one of the most intensively studied areas of vertebrate anatomy and physiology[2].

Together, the hearing and equilibrium structures of the inner ear make up what is collectively known as the *labyrinth*. Despite what is often depicted in images of the inner ear (see Figure 1.2), the labyrinth organs are not free-standing structures; rather, they are tunnels that pass through the deep portions of the temporal bone (Figure 1.1). These tunnels are lined with membranes that serve to contain the specialized fluid known as endolymph that is contained within the labyrinth. As we will discuss, it is the movement of this fluid within the vestibular portion of the labyrinth that provides much of our ability to detect certain motions of the head.

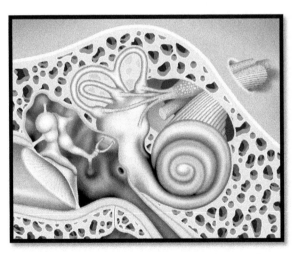

Figure 1.1 The labyrinth system does not consist of free-standing structures but rather a group of hollowed-out areas of the temporal bone that form a series of cavities and tunnels

Any involvement of the labyrinth specific to the symptoms of MdDS has not yet been clearly outlined. However, given the associated symptoms of unsteadiness and 'rocking' that often accompanies MdDS, there is likely some degree of interplay between MdDS and the labyrinth, particularly the vestibular portion of the labyrinth. Although the cochlea, a snail-shaped organ responsible for processing sound, is a major component of the labyrinth, there is relatively little direct involvement with hearing in MdDS. Therefore, we'll focus our efforts predominantly on the vestibular system, given its more likely link to the symptoms that commonly occur in response to MdDS.

The vestibular system itself consists of two separate structures that are designed to detect movement of the head (Figure 1.2). When the head moves in a particular direction, these structures send their corresponding signals along a neural pathway to the brain where the interpretation of the signal occurs in order to determine head movement. Because there are separate 'detection' and 'interpretation' components, the labyrinth is referred to as the *peripheral* vestibular system while the brain – responsible for interpreting signals from the labyrinth – is described as the *central* vestibular system.

While each component of the vestibular system does perform independently, they are also highly dependent upon each other. Outlining the uniqueness of the two systems is important, especially in light of the fact that certain vestibular-based conditions may be considered as 'central' in origin while others are classified as peripheral-based disorders.

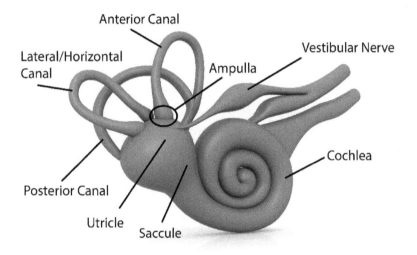

Figure 1.2. The labyrinth system is comprised of several individual organs including the cochlea, vestibule, and semicircular canals.

Peripheral Vestibular anatomy

Our body detects movement and motion through a complicated mix of inputs involving our feet, joints, and even our vision. While pressure receptors within our feet and joint-angle receptors embedded within our limbs are certainly valuable in terms of their role in motion detection, we will limit our scope of motion detection to those components involved with the peripheral vestibular system itself. Again, it is important to stress that the true cause of MdDS may involve several different body systems; however, because MdDS is suspected to be linked to the vestibular system (either peripheral or central), we'll focus predominantly on describing the makeup of the vestibular system.

Five independent structures are involved in our peripheral vestibular system's ability to detect head motion. The first two structures are housed within an organ called the vestibule, a 3-5mm wide structure located between the cochlea and semicircular canals. The vestibule itself contains two very important components called the *saccule* and the *utricle* that are responsible for detecting motion that occurs in a linear direction (i.e. forward/backward, up/down, side-to-side). Activities such as running, walking, standing up, or even riding in an elevator are capable of being detected by the saccule and the utricle, both of which have thousands of small crystals embedded within them to help detect inertia. Because the saccule and utricle house these small crystals known as *otoliths*, both structures are known as the "otolith organs".

In addition to the saccule and utricle, the remainder of the vestibular portion of the inner ear is comprised of three canals called semicircular canals that form loops through the temporal bone. These canals detect *angular* motion, the kind when you shake your head 'yes' or 'no'. The semicircular canals also play a very important role in ensuring that our eyes can stay on a fixed spot or target even while our head is moving due to a unique link between the inner ear and eyes in a specialized reflex that we will discuss later in this chapter.

Now, we'll look at each of these structures in more depth so as to gain a better understanding of how each is involved in our ability to detect motion and maintain equilibrium.

Saccule

The saccule is a portion of the vestibule responsible for detecting vertical motion of the head (and with vertical movement of the head typically comes movement of the body as well). For example, jumping up and down or riding in an elevator are activities that stimulate the motion sensors within the saccule. Inside the saccule is a structure called the *macula sacculi*, a vertically-oriented organ that houses a two- to three-millimeter area comprised of sensory hair cells responsible for sensing head motion. The ends of these hair cells extend horizontally into the middle of the vestibule and are covered by a gelatinous layer, over which is a fibrous structure called the otolithic membrane. It is this otolithic membrane that contains the small calcium-based crystals known by a variety of names including *statoconia, otoconia,* and the aforementioned *otolith.*

Because it is embedded with otoliths, the otolithic membrane is heavier than the material surrounding it (Figure 1.3). Therefore, when the body moves somewhat quickly in a vertical plane such as occurs when jumping, gravity pulls the otoliths downward the same way as a leafy branch might bend when you swing it upward. The weight of the otoliths causes hair cells that extend into the otolithic membrane to bend in response to the linear motion. This in turn causes those nerve cells to send a signal to the brain that is interpreted as vertical movement of the head.

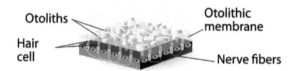

Figure 1.3. Otoliths embedded within the otolithic membrane interact with gravity to trigger hair cells to bend, thereby initiating a signal to the brain specific to head movement.

Utricle

The utricle has an almost identical makeup as the saccule but exhibits a slightly different orientation and function. The utricle is larger than the saccule and is responsible for detecting when our head moves in a horizontal plane. Such movements – which occur with

forward, backward, or side-to-side motion of the head –
occur when walking, running, or even riding in a car.
Like the saccule, the utricle contains a macula called the
macula utriculi. In contrast to the saccule's vertically-
oriented macula, the macula utriculi is positioned
horizontally and embedded with hair cells that are
oriented vertically. The macula utriculi detects motion
similar to that of the macula sacculi in that the hair cells
are covered with a gelatinous layer which is in turn
overlaid with a gel-like membrane embedded with
otoliths. Horizontal motion of the head generates inertia
that then causes the embedded hair cells to bend and send
a signal to the brain indicative of the direction of head
movement.

Semicircular Canals

Along with the vestibule's saccule and utricle
structures, there are three semicircular canals of the inner
ear's labyrinth network that make up the remainder of
the peripheral vestibular system. As mentioned earlier,
the semicircular canals are not true bony structures
themselves; rather, they exist as 'tunnels' or canals
through the temporal bone. Thin membranes line the
bone-encased semicircular canals and serve to contain
fluid known as endolymph that is found throughout the
labyrinth system. Rotational or 'angular' motions of the

head – such as occurs when turning the head back and forth at a tennis match – cause this endolymph to move within the canals in a process that we will discuss shortly. Because angular movement does not generate enough inertia within the inner ear to act upon the saccule or utricle, the design of the semicircular canals allow them to detect this angular motion as the endolymph flows across specialized sensors within each canal. The brain then interprets the signal from these sensors to establish the direction of head movement.

There are three independent semicircular canals – the anterior, posterior, and horizontal canals. The orientation of the three canals positions them at right angles to each other which in turn allows all head motions to be detected. This design can be imagined by thinking of a corner of a cube – each of the three sides of the cube represents a different plane of movement similar to how any angular movement of the head can be detected by one or more of the semicircular canals.

So how does the movement of fluid within the semicircular canals actually result in the brain being able to detect head motion? Angular motion is detected due to endolymph passing over a specialized organ within each canal called the *cupula*. Movement of the head in an angular motion (i.e. shaking the head 'no', nodding the head, etc.) causes movement of endolymph, which in turn flows across hair cells that move in response to the flow of endolymph. The cupula is located within the canal itself, at each end of the semicircular canals in a bulged-out area called the *ampulla* (see Figure 1.2). Hair cells within the ampulla extend into the cupula, a gelatinous layer over the hair cells that extends into each semicircular canal.

Let's look at this process in a little more detail. When a person moves his or her head, the endolymph moves within the semicircular canal in response to the head movement. As the fluid moves, it flows around the cupula (Figure 1.4). This in turn causes the cupula bends in response to the fluid moving over it. This causes hair cells immediately under the cupula to also bend, the same way we earlier described that tree branch bending if its leafy end were placed into flowing water. This bending of the hair cells then sends a signal to the brain which is interpreted as motion corresponding to the actual direction of head movement.

These events occurring within the semicircular canals are important to understand, as they are thought to play a role in dizziness. As far back as the 1960s, researchers believed that conditions such as benign paroxysmal positional vertigo (BPPV) – which triggers bouts of vertigo, nystagmus (i.e. rapid eye motion), and unsteadiness – resulted from otoliths pressing against the cupula within the semicircular canal[3]. Even back then, this activity was suspected of increasing the cupula's sensitivity to the fluid motion, in turn generating the symptoms associated with conditions such as BPPV.

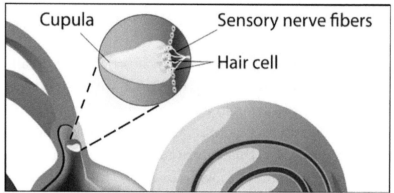

Figure 1.4. Near the end of each semicircular canal, the ampulla houses the sensitive cupula organ which is responsible for detecting movement of fluid within the respective semicircular canal

Non-vestibular perception of balance

Besides the vestibular system, there are two other primary sources of input to help us maintain our balance as well as provide feedback specific to voluntary movement. These systems include visual feedback – particularly useful in what is known as 'spatial orientation' – or the ability to recognize our body's position within the environment around it – and our somatosensory system which consists of receptors that provide feedback specific to joint position, muscle force, and foot pressure, among others. While it is not known how MdDS is affected by any or all of these systems, the propensity for impaired balance in response to MdDS makes it necessary for us to at least introduce ourselves to these additional input sources. While the underlying issue behind MdDS may lie in the brain's ability to interpret input received by these systems, a basic understanding of their role in our ability to maintain balance is warranted.

While all three (vestibular, visual, somatosensory) systems exist independently, they intermix quite a bit in order to provide us feedback specific to our body's position and balance. To outline this, let's look at an example. Take, for instance, a setting in which you are walking in a large cluttered warehouse looking for an item. Most likely you give little thought to any of these vestibular systems as you can clearly see where you are going, thereby suppressing any input from your feet or limbs as there is no suspicious surface or obstacle to prevent you from walking normally. Suddenly, as you turn a corner to head to the exit, the lights suddenly go out and leave you in complete darkness. No one in their right mind will continue walking at the same speed in an unfamiliar area as it's an almost guaranteed recipe for injury, and our body refuses to willingly allow that to happen. Instead, we alter our gait to take shorter, more controlled steps. Perhaps we slowly slide our foot forward, paying attention to each step specific to how the underlying surface feels as well as if there is anything in our way. We might reach our arms out, feeling for any obstructive object that might hinder our path to the exit. In the right situation, it becomes clear that we need each of our sensory inputs despite the fact that we often forget that they are even there.

Because of the interplay of the three balance systems, the brain is tasked with the responsibility of figuring out which one to pay the most attention towards. If, for example, you are sitting still in a chair, there is very little movement going on at your joints or within your head. In such a case, your visual feedback likely makes it clear that you are stationary and there is no pressing need to keep the balance systems alert. However, the visual system can also fail you. Have you ever pulled into a parking spot right at the moment that the car next to you backs out of theirs? This phenomenon tricks the visual input system to the point that you most likely tense your muscles and quickly focus on another visual source in order to 'orient' yourself to the fact that you are indeed *not* moving. This, in effect, is one example of how the brain can misinterpret feedback.

Another example can highlight the event of improper balance-based feedback. Being on a boat or airplane is notorious for causing this because we see and feel a solid surface when on the boat deck or seated in our aisle, but that surface is in turn placed in a highly unstable environment when on the water or in the air. In other words, though we are directly connected to a stable chair or standing on a solid deck, the support for that –

the boat or airplane – is moving in quite an unstable environment itself. Instead of a linear-type motion (i.e. motion that involves only one direction such as when walking), passive motion on a boat or airplane involves multiple directions such as side-to-side combined with up and down (and maybe even a little front and back mixed in). In some cases, there may even be a bit of angular motion that is detected by the semicircular canal thrown in as well. Suddenly, our body's balance-detection systems are sensing inertia-based feedback from the motion of the waves or the rocking of the plane, yet also trying to figure out why there might be no movement in your joints while you are sitting in your chair. This in turn confuses our brain into processing why we seem stable yet for some reason we are receiving 'unstable' feedback sensations. Moreover, when this conflict occurs within the bowels of the ship or when the window shades are closed on an airplane it can become particularly problematic as there is no true point of reference on which your brain can visually focus in order to 'reset' itself.

While we have directed our attention in this chapter primarily at the vestibular system's role in maintaining balance, there is no question that all three systems (vestibular, visual, somatosensory) are involved in providing feedback. This is certainly not to say that the vestibular system is utilized more or that it is more prioritized over the others. We could easily venture into a discussion of baroreceptors, the cervicocolic reflex, or the vestibulocolic reflex, but these systems are not quite as simple to outline and are based on neural signaling and interaction with the brain which is not as well understood as the vestibular system. Nevertheless, I would like to close out this chapter with a couple of aspects related closely to vision and balance, specifically vertigo as well as the vestibulo-ocular reflex, or 'VOR', as I think that the role of vision coupled with vestibular input is important to understand from the context of MdDS. The VOR is highly involved in the symptom of vertigo, and whereas it has been suggested that MdDS is a *form* of vertigo[4, 5], we will take a closer look at vertigo itself. Whereas the principles of vertigo may be involved with MdDS, in the next section we'll briefly outline vertigo in order to allow you to grasp the basic aspects of this annoying symptom.

Vertigo

Vertigo is the sensation of movement when in fact no movement is occurring. It is important to understand that vertigo is a symptom – not an actual medical condition; therefore, expecting a cure for vertigo is effectively the same as asking your physician to cure pain. What is likely meant is that you want a cure for what is *causing* the vertigo. Vertigo itself is largely thought to result from events occurring within the inner ear; therefore, medical conditions that trigger vertigo – such as BPPV – often originate from within the inner ear. However, many vertigo-inducing conditions are not well understood and are suspected to involve a complex interaction between the brain (i.e. 'central' type vertigo) and the inner ear (i.e. 'peripheral' vertigo).

As a patient of a balance-related condition, it is important to understand that vertigo has several possible sources, and no one event or structure has been established as a primary cause for vertigo. However, researchers have largely narrowed peripheral vertigo down to the semicircular canals, saccule, or utricle, while central vertigo is typically associated with either the brainstem or the vestibulocochlear nerve[6]. When functioning normally, the inner ear structures send signals to the brain in a coordinated pattern from the left and right ear. However, an imbalance of these vestibular inputs – such as can occur when one of our two vestibular systems is not performing correctly – leads to uncoordinated information being transmitted to the brain, in turn triggering events such as nystagmus or vertigo to occur. This imbalanced signal can occur due to disruption anywhere along the neural pathway that stretches from the inner ear to the brain.

Again, there is no specific structure or area that triggers vertigo across all patients. Therefore, vertigo can arise from multiple causes and conditions. For example, patients experiencing migraine (a specific type of headache) sometimes experience vertigo similar to patients who have a disorder specific to the vestibule of the inner ear. Vertigo can even originate from outside of the skull, such as can occur in patients who suffer from degenerating intervertebral discs, a condition known as 'cervical vertigo'[7].

One confounding issue that medical professionals have in establishing vertigo is that patients often lump it in with dizziness. Both vertigo and dizziness are indeed similar in their effects given that each can make you as the patient feel unsteady. One recommended way to separate the two conditions is to outline whether you feel 'lightheaded' or whether you feel as though the world is spinning around you. Generally, a spinning sensation is more characteristic of vertigo, while lightheadedness is typically associated with dizziness[8]. Certainly, feeling lightheaded is a common complaint with MdDS while a true 'spinning' vertigo-type sensation is rather infrequent. Therefore, as a patient of MdDS it is important to clarify whether you are going through a type of 'dizziness' or whether you are experiencing vertigo.

So what exactly causes the sensation of vertigo? Physiologically speaking, vertigo is largely due to a link between the inner ear and the eyes. While this may seem to be a somewhat odd link, the interconnection between our ears and eyes plays a vital role in our daily function even though we may not recognize it (until there is a problem!). To outline this role, we'll next discuss the vestibulo-ocular reflex (VOR) and how it coordinates interaction between the ear and eye. The brain's processing of the VOR may play a role in the symptoms associated with MdDS[9]; therefore, I think it's essential that we outline the VOR in order to help you understand the potential involvement that this reflex may have in MdDS.

The vestibulo-ocular reflex (VOR)

Although our eyes have an independent function specific to providing our sense of vision, they are in fact intimately connected with the inner ear. This interaction plays an important role in our ability to maintain balance as well as to maintain acuity when we are moving. To illustrate how important your vision is for aiding in your balance, walk quickly from a bright room into a very dark one. You'll probably find that you are initially timid and a little bit unsteady, which will likely improve once your eyes adjust to the darkness. Now, jump up and down a few times and notice how your vision of the area around you is still quite clear and steady – a stark contrast from watching a video that was recorded on a camera held while jumping. The ability to maintain this smooth field of vision even while engaged in strenuous activity such as jumping is because of the intricate link between the vestibular system and movement of the eyes. The link between our inner ear and eyes is known as the *vestibulo-ocular reflex'*, or "VOR". We won't go deep into the details of how the VOR works, but we'll take a moment to describe a general overview of the reflex as it can relate to a few expected symptoms of MdDS.

The interconnection between your vestibular system and eyes is what allows you to maintain a smooth, non-jumpy field of vision while running or when riding on a bumpy road. This smooth control happens because the vestibular system has a degree of control over the muscles of the eyes through the VOR such that your eyes can remain fixed on an object even though your head position may be moving. The VOR reflex has the task of trying to ensure that an image or object remains stable on your retina in order to allow for proper processing by the brain[10]. Without the VOR, every time your head moves, you would consciously need to readjust your eye position back to the object you are looking at. With the VOR, however, your vestibular system is able to detect the speed of your head motion and automatically control the muscles in your eye so that your gaze easily remains fixed on the object. This reflex also works well when driving, as every time you hit a bump or turn a corner your eyes are subconsciously controlled by the VOR rather than jumping all around while trying to manually reposition – which would certainly be a problem when operating a vehicle!

When the VOR is working correctly you don't even know that it's there. But when there is a disruption to the system – such as occurs in response to several vestibular-related diseases – the VOR becomes impaired and can lead to uncontrolled movements such as the aforementioned nystagmus. Consequently, an affected patient is not able to coordinate their eye movements with the movements of their head. This can lead to jumpy or blurry vision, likely occurring most often when the head is moving or the patient's body is in motion. Another condition that can result is *oscillopsia,* a condition in which objects in the field of vision appear to float around even though they are in fact stationary, due in large part to the muscles of the eye being unable to keep the eye adequately fixed on one object.

Additional visual problems can occur when a person with a faulty VOR tries to follow movement or read text on paper or a computer screen, a process known as *tracking.* With a mal-functioning VOR not allowing for smooth eye movement such as that required to follow a thrown ball or read printed text, it can be difficult for the patient to make the smooth eye motions needed to properly intake visual information (i.e. identify and process the written words). This can in turn cause quite a disruption to a patient's daily life, as trying to maintain normal function without a well-established link between our eyes and our ears can be quite difficult. The VOR helps make our ability to gather visual input a relatively simple process, but unfortunately this link between our eyes and ears requires us to pay the price of having visual disturbances such as vertigo or nystagmus when our vestibular system is malfunctioning.

Conclusion

Clearly, the inner ear consists of highly intricate and complex structures. Without a properly functioning vestibular system, our ability to maintain posture, recognize our movements, and sense positional changes can be extremely difficult. The intent of this chapter was to provide an overview of those structural components of the inner ear involved in vestibular-type disorders that can affect a patient's balance or equilibrium. In addition, we touched on several physiological processes that can occur in conjunction with MdDS. Understand that what we covered in this chapter is indeed quite broad in scope; there is in fact much, much more that we could discuss at a deeper level. However, as I stated in the introduction my focus is to keep this book oriented as a guide for MdDS patients rather than serving as a medical textbook. What you will hopefully find is that as you continue to read subsequent chapters, the detailed information we have discussed here becomes more relevant to you given that you better understand the various anatomy and physiology of the inner ear. Next, we'll look more closely at two symptoms related to MdDS, specifically dizziness and seasickness.

Chapter 2 – Dizziness and sea sickness

UNDERSTANDING THE BODY'S balance systems is beneficial in being able to recognize the underlying structures and physiology that may be involved in MdDS. Whereas imbalance and unsteadiness are characteristics of MdDS, having a better understanding of the physiology of how our body maintains its equilibrium can provide you the patient with a more clear understanding of the complexity of how these systems work together to allow us to maintain our posture. Now, we'll focus our attention on two conditions – dizziness and seasickness – that are associated with MdDS so as to outline the similarities as well as the differences between the conditions. While seasickness is not commonly associated with MdDS, I feel that it would be beneficial to discuss seasickness given that it shares some of the same origins of MdDS, particularly in that it is caused by passive motion such as what occurs while on a ship. Therefore, this chapter will focus on outlining just what dizziness and seasickness are as well as discussing the many potential causes of each. In understanding the causes of dizziness and seasickness, it can help patients separate out MdDS from these other related conditions.

Dizziness

Dizziness is a symptom, much like pain. And it can be a costly symptom, with current medical expense estimates of up to $50 billion per year resulting from dizziness[11]. Because dizziness is a symptom that must be reported and described by the patient, we do not have a good test that can measure the type or degree of dizziness that a patient experiences[12]. Whereas there are no tests for dizziness, patients are typically left to describe their symptoms, which itself can be difficult to do[13]. It is also important that patients are able to differentiate dizziness from vertigo. As we discussed in the prior chapter, vertigo is the perception of movement when no movement is actually occurring. If you've ever had vertigo, you are familiar with the sensation that makes it seem as though the room is spinning, or that you are spinning within the room. Dizziness is not vertigo, though, and does not involve perceived motion as much as a sensation that one's balance is 'off' or that they feel lightheaded.

Much like pain, dizziness can come in many forms and can be the result of many different causes. Dizziness is relatively common, with up to 8% of people reporting dizziness at some point in their lifetime[14]. Unfortunately, dizziness does not have a clear definition[15], likely because it comes in many forms in much the same way that pain has many potential forms. For example, pain can be achy, sharp, or dull and can arise from a joint, bone, nerve impingement, or tissue trauma, amongst other causes. Likewise, dizziness can occur in response to dehydration, positional changes (e.g. going around a corner), standing up from a seated position, or perhaps from an ear infection. Consequences of these events can be revealed in physical manifestations, as it is expected that a patient complaining of dizziness generally has some sort of issue that affects their posture and/or gait[12]. Recognizing the various causes as well as effects of dizziness can help differentiate any dizziness reported with MdDS from the many other forms.

Causes of dizziness

As mentioned, 'dizziness' as a symptom can come in many forms. Some of the various conditions that could be intermixed with the general understanding of the term 'dizziness' could include nausea, vertigo, lightheadedness, imbalance, or unsteadiness[15]. Because of these various causes, up to 35% of the population is said to experience some degree of dizziness during their life[16], and dizziness is one of the most common reasons for visits to a physician[17]. Up to 12% of people in the United States are thought to have experienced dizziness in the past 12 months[18], and the percent of people affected gets much higher amongst an older population[16]. However, it's also known that up to half of individuals who experience dizziness do not seek medical attention[19], suggesting that the true number of people affected by dizziness is actually much higher.

Dizziness associated with the vestibular system typically influences a patient's sense of balance when moving his or her head[15]. In fact, some of the most common causes of dizziness that require a medical evaluation are localized to the inner ear, as one study reported that BPPV was the most common cause (33.9%), followed by phobic postural vertigo (21.4%), Ménière's disease (20%), vestibular neuronitis/labyrinthitis (8.1%), and vestibular migraine (4.1%)[17]. When dizziness is of a vestibular source, the issue typically lies with either one or both balance organs (e.g. semicircular canals, vestibule), the vestibular nerve that carries the signal from the balance organs to the brain, or the brain's ability to process the signals[20]. Initially, a significant degree of vertigo or imbalance will likely occur in response to diminished activity within the inner ear, at least until the brain adequately adjusts to the diminished function, which may include those times that the patient is not moving[20]. Hours or days later, the patient may begin to experience a lessened degree of symptoms when stationary, but still may continue to have similar issues when movement occurs. Overcoming this phase of vestibular deficit takes longer and often requires specific exercises to help the brain adapt to the diminished vestibular function[20]. In addition, a patient will likely have a smoother recovery if the dizziness only occurs in one ear[20]. If both inner-ear vestibular mechanisms are compromised, recovery will take longer and the patient will most likely experience symptoms even during normal activity[20].

As discussed, vestibular issues are not the only cause for dizziness, as patients who feel imbalance after moving to a standing position may have cardiac or circulatory issues rather than a vestibular-based source of dizziness. For example, dizziness can occur in patients with low blood pressure who cannot maintain adequate blood flow to the brain when moving from a lying or seated position to standing[21]. Other instances include dizziness that occurs when the eyes are moved in absence of head movement, which suggests an anxiety-related source[15]. Because MdDS is most likely related to dizziness of a vestibular or balance-sensory origin, we will not discuss these cardiac or anxiety-related causes.

Impact of dizziness

It's one thing to have dizziness, but it's another issue if the dizziness affects an individual's daily life. As would be expected, dizziness can impact daily activities to the point that patients will avoid leaving the house and may even require sick leave from work[19]. Depending on the degree of dizziness experienced by the patient, he or she may end up with decreases in quality of life, social life, and/or an ability to perform normal daily tasks[16], which can end up inviting feelings of helplessness as well as result in a patient isolating him or herself from others. In addition, as dizziness is somewhat related to one's ability to maintain balance, experiencing dizziness can increase the risk of falls which can unfortunately cause injury and result in significant medical costs[22]. The injury and subsequent medical expense can in turn contribute heavily to the resulting decrease in quality of life that dizziness can bring[23].

Treatment of dizziness

To treat a patient's dizziness it is first essential to understand the source of the dizziness. For example, if a patient simply has an ear infection there is no benefit to giving them blood pressure medication as a means to improve their dizziness, as the ear infection is the true source. Therefore, a simple dose or two of antibiotics may indeed clear their dizziness symptoms within a day or two. If the cause of the dizziness is vestibular in nature, it is essential that the particular vestibular condition is identified. For example, if the patient is experiencing dizziness associated with BPPV, a relatively simple 'canalith repositioning' procedure can effectively fix the dizziness. Other vestibular-related dizziness from causes such as Ménière's disease or vestibular neuritis may be improved through dietary modifications (e.g. low-sodium diet), undergoing balance training therapy, or use of certain prescription (e.g. triptans) or non-prescription (e.g. dimenhydrinate) drugs. Unfortunately, though, some vestibular-related dizziness does not respond well to treatment and may ultimately require significant adjustments on the part of the patient such as using assistance (e.g. cane) when walking or requiring transportation help.

Seasickness

Being dizzy typically involves a feeling of lightheadedness and may affect an individual's stability but does not manifest itself much past that. Seasickness, on the other hand, may induce additional symptoms. As a medical condition, seasickness goes by many names:

motion sickness, travel sickness, car sickness, or its more professional name of *morbus nauticus*. Seasickness is typically the result of travel on ships or boats, airplanes, or cars, but can also occur in response to visual stimuli such as movies or video games. Symptoms generally include nausea, sweating, and paleness, among others, and may eventually induce vomiting. For most people, seasickness is quite an unpleasant experience but is usually transient in nature, typically stopping at or soon after the end of the trigger (e.g. boat travel).

The underlying cause of seasickness is not known, nor is it known why some people are more at risk of seasickness than others. The 'sensory conflict' theory suggests that in affected individuals, the visual, vestibular, and sensory inputs are in conflict, thereby confusing the brain as to what motion it should respond[24]. In other words, while one might feel as though they are standing on a stable boat surface, the vestibular system receives input that the patient is moving up and down, thereby confusing the brain as to what is actually occurring. Alternatively, an idea known as the *postural control theory* suggests that motion sickness results from an inability to properly maintain adequate posture in response to the passive forces placed upon the body[24]. Various other theories exist that attempt to explain the cause of seasickness, though none have yet identified the true source of the symptoms.

Treatment of seasickness

There are several viable options for treating seasickness. During an acute attack, establishing a visual path with the horizon can help many patients, particularly if the initial attack began when the patient did not have any external views such as might happen if being 'below deck' while on the water. Another treatment option involves 'habituation', which entails repeated exposure to a seasickness-inducing trigger in an attempt to desensitize the patient to the offending motion. Research has shown that such training can have lasting effects for affected patients that can extend months or more after the training ends[25].

Alternative treatments for motion sickness include transcutaneous electrical nerve stimulation, stress reduction, and pharmacologic intervention[24]. Most drug-based therapies target either histamine or the vestibular/vomiting control areas in the body[24]. Therefore, antihistamines (e.g. meclizine) and anticholinergic drugs such as scopolamine are often used to combat seasickness. Drug therapies have been shown to reduce symptoms, but they do not generally prevent or cure seasickness[24]. Furthermore, notable side effects such as drowsiness are commonly associated with pharmacological treatment of seasickness, which may be problematic for those such as pilots who require alertness.

Natural remedies for seasickness such as herbs/spices or supplements show some promise for abating the effects of seasickness and could be considered to have fewer side effects[24]. Acupressure bands, however, have not shown favorable results for preventing seasickness[24], but have been shown beneficial for preventing nausea of various origins[26].

Conclusion

Because MdDS can have a dizziness component and is induced through passive motion similar to what can induce seasickness, I felt it was relevant to briefly discuss the characteristics of each. Gaining a general understanding of the mechanisms involved with dizziness and seasickness can help outline some of the complexities of MdDS even though there are indeed separate and unique aspects of each. If MdDS is a diagnosis you have received yourself, there is a likely chance that you are experiencing some degree of vestibular or proprioceptive-related dizziness rather than any type related to a cardiac source. Now that we have covered the body's balance systems as well as general aspects of dizziness and seasickness, you have a firm overview toward understanding some of the inner workings involved with MdDS. Therefore, we will next dive into MdDS as a medical condition itself, drawing on what we have discussed specific to the body's balance controls in order to help outline aspects such as the suspected causes, the involved symptoms, and who is affected.

Chapter 3: What is MdDS?

Vestibular-type disorders seem to have received a sudden surge in attention over the past 30 or so years. Other, more prominent conditions such as stroke, concussion, or even diabetes have been thoroughly researched for over a century or more and therefore have a much broader understanding as well as more numerous and directed treatment options. On the one hand, it can be frustrating to learn that a condition such as MdDS has not yet received clear diagnostic criteria as a result of its relative 'newness' in the medical arena. Yet, at the same time it's encouraging to note that the condition has gained traction in the area of medical research over the past couple of decades, thereby providing hope for advanced treatment options and perhaps even a cure. Still, for those suffering from the effects of MdDS a cure remains elusive, thereby leaving only hope for continued research that may lead to treatments capable of providing relief from the ongoing misery that can be brought about by this disease. Next, we'll use the information discussed in the previous chapters to focus our efforts directly on MdDS in order to outline just who is affected, the associated symptoms, and suspected causes of MdDS.

MdDS Terminology

The term *mal de debarquement* can be translated literally into 'bad disembarkment'. In the medical literature, the condition of MdDS has been discussed using several terms including Mal de Debarquement, sea legs, or rocking dizziness[27]. In the last 50 or so years, the term *Mal de Debarquement Syndrome* has gained a foothold[4]. Still, there is a bit of conflict in the literature between what comprises a normal or expected residual effect of motion after getting off a ship versus what is considered problematic. For example, some researchers claim that dizziness occurring within the first 48 hours after disembarking a vessel is considered transient in nature and thereby not indicative of the more problematic MdDS unless it lasts for three days or more, at which point it is considered persistent MdDS[28]. Others have suggested that when the associated symptoms disappear within one month, the condition is considered as Mal de Debarquement, while symptoms that persist longer than a month warrants the term Mal de Debarquement Syndrome[29]. Some other terms you might read in the medical literature include motion-triggered (MT) MdDS, which is classified as that type brought about by exposure to motion, and spontaneous-onset MdDS, which is specific to MdDS that appears without the prior trigger of motion[30].

For the purposes of this book, we will focus on using the term *Mal de Debarquement Syndrome*, represented as MdDS, so as to differentiate between the chronic condition and the more commonly experienced yet shorter-lasting Mal de Debarquement.

A brief history of MdDS

Seasickness has probably been occurring as long as humans have traveled on the water. Most likely, given our lack of gills or webbed extremities, our body evolved to tackle the challenges posed on land and left behind any residual association with the sea. Our ability to conquer the water, though, occurred in part due to our ability to navigate the seas. This in turn brought about a new sensation to our body, one that involved our walking on a solid surface that was itself made somewhat unstable as it traversed through the water.

Hippocrates may have been the first to recognize our body's struggle with a life on the sea, as his early description of *nausea* came in part from the word "naus", which is Greek for 'ship'. He was the first to record that being on a ship was responsible for causing motion disruption to the body[31]. Much later, in the late 1700s, Erasmus Darwin made note of individuals complaining of feeling as though they were still on the water even though they had returned to land[32]. It's not known whether he was referring to seasickness or some degree of MdDS, but it's certainly possible that he was referencing at least some degree of MdDS, much like how in the late 1800s sailors were often reported to have an unsteady gait when returning from a stormy voyage[33].

Not much mention occurred in the medical literature over the next 100 years until researchers Brown and Baloh reported in 1987 on six individuals with a conspicuous condition that arose after disembarking from a ship[34]. This publication, along with growing interest in the vestibular system, finally helped spur directed research toward MdDS as a medical condition that has continued to grow over the past two decades. Evidence of recent interest in MdDS within the medical literature is made clear by reports that over two-thirds of all MdDS-related research has been published since 2005, with much of this research focusing on experiment-based studies rather than case reports that were more commonly utilized for MdDS in prior years[35].

Who is affected by MdDS

Because MdDS is so new – and quite rare – as a recognized medical condition, we don't yet have a wealth of data that can reveal consistencies as to the type of person affected. What we do know, however, is that the highest reported group affected by MdDS is middle-aged women[36]. This fact was made glaringly clear while researching this book and coming across a study designed to look at personality traits in MdDS and finding the following statement: *Fifty-four women and one man have participated in the MdDS research studies to date*[37]. Nevertheless, males do experience MdDS, but they account for no more than one-fourth of patients[27] and have been reported to comprise as few as 10% of MdDS cases[29].

Specific to age, both males and females typically develop MdDS in their 40s or 50s[29]. Unfortunately, the incidence rate of MdDS (i.e. how many new cases occur per year) is not currently known. However, one study conducted at a neurotology clinic reported that 1.3% of patients were classified as having MdDS[38].

What is MdDS?

Unlike several other vestibular-based conditions, MdDS is not common and is in fact considered to be a rare neurological condition[39]. This rarity, combined with its relatively short history as a medical disorder, likely contributes to why patients report seeing from 5 - 19 medical professionals before receiving a proper diagnosis[29, 40]. Despite the prominent symptoms that are inherent to MdDS, patients typically find that their inner-ear function is normal and imaging studies (e.g. CT, MRI) indicate no abnormalities[34].

As a medical condition, MdDS has been described as the sensation of persistent perception of self-motion that occurs after a period of passive motion[39]. Passive motion is motion that occurs without active input from the individual; therefore, riding on a boat would induce passive motion due to the action of the waves on the boat, while a person who is walking or running would be considered to be inducing active motion. In keeping with this definition, the most common cause of MdDS is travel on water via boat or ship, which is to say that MdDS typically occurs when a patient is exposed to an extended period of a particular type of passive motion. However, travel on water is not the only source, as air travel has been known to cause MdDS as well[41].

It is important to point out that MdDS is *typically* caused by exposure to passive motion. Researchers have found that a small percentage of patients are afflicted with MdDS without having first been exposed to passive motion such as would be brought about by a ship or airplane. Patients who fall into this category are said to suffer from a subtype of MdDS referred to by some as 'spontaneous' or 'other-onset' MdDS, whereby symptoms started either spontaneously or after some event such as a surgery, childbirth, or a stressful event[42].

The initiation of MdDS symptoms after ongoing exposure to passive motion would suggest that MdDS is in fact a balance disorder. While this idea makes sense, one inherent problem in identifying MdDS as a balance disorder is that a good proportion of patients actually feel worse when lying down[4]. As pointed out by researchers, logic would hold that if MdDS were indeed a balance-related disorder – including one involving the brain's processing of balance inputs – eliminating the need to maintain balance by lying down would, in theory, make the patient feel better. With MdDS, however, improvement in symptoms when lying down is not consistent across patients and therefore lends more questions as to the true underlying cause of MdDS.

As has been mentioned, the specific cause of MdDS has not yet been determined. This is not to say, though, that a potential cause has not been narrowed down, as scientists have been able to reveal certain aspects that allow us to better understand the possible mechanisms behind the symptoms associated with MdDS. Structurally speaking, for example, researchers have shown that MdDS patients exhibit altered gray matter in areas of the brain responsible for visual and vestibular signal processing, along with gray matter alterations in other areas of the brain as well[43]. Both the location of these changes in the brain as well as the vestibular-related function of this particular area of tissue is significant as it lends physical evidence to explain the rocking sensation associated with MdDS, as well as why patients often experience a reduction in symptoms when re-exposed to the original source of their MdDS symptoms.

A separate study found similar brain-related changes in MdDS patients. Specifically, hyper-metabolic activity in the left entorhinal cortex and amygdala areas of the brain along with a hypo-metabolism (i.e. reduced activity) in several other areas[44]. Furthermore, it was reported that MdDS subjects exhibited increased neural connectivity between both the entorhinal cortex and amygdala portions of the brain with the posterior visual and vestibular processing areas within the brain. In short, these findings clarify that the brain can exhibit unique activity in MdDS patients. If you are interested in the detailed findings of these studies, the articles cited can be found online and provide much more detail specific to how each affected area of the brain may contribute to the symptoms of MdDS.

Based on findings from these and other studies, researchers have proposed a few theories that attempt to decipher the cause of MdDS. Unfortunately, it quickly becomes clear that even in our age of medical advancements, the fact that theories are still our best indicator of the cause of a medical condition helps illustrate the underlying complexity of MdDS.

The associated theories behind the cause of MdDS are based upon the concept of *neuroplasticity*[41], which focuses on the ability of the brain to change how it handles certain neural processes. In one theory, researchers have suggested that MdDS may result from an over-synchronization of networks within the brain that may become 'tricked' into associating with the passive motion that originally caused a patient's symptoms[35]. A second theory proposes that the VOR may be involved in MdDS such that multi-sensory inputs may 'throw off' the VOR during passive motion environments such as what occurs on a boat[9]. Rehabilitation designed around this second theory attempts to 'refocus' the VOR through the use of visual stimuli. A third proposed theory suggests that there is a specific motion capable of causing MdDS that involves the combined motions of pitch, vertical motion, and roll[45]. Support for this theory was provided when symptoms of MdDS disappeared after specific treatment designed to counter these motions.

Certainly, each of these theories has a scientific basis, and it is also entirely likely that all theories are on track towards establishing an as-yet undetermined cause of MdDS. Without question, more research is needed to better define the true cause of MdDS, particularly because – as one researcher noted – ship cruises continue to be a popular vacation choice[45]. This inevitably means that individuals will most likely continue to be afflicted by MdDS, thereby emphasizing the need for effective treatment.

Symptoms of Mal de Debarquement

Up to 75% of people who get off of a ship report some degree of unsteadiness in what is called land-sickness[46]. It is this land sickness that is classified by some as transient mal de debarquement. Not unexpectedly, individuals prone to land-sickness are typically susceptible to seasickness as well; however, what might be considered quite odd is that individuals affected by MdDS are not generally prone to seasickness. This may have to do with the fact that seasickness starts *during* passive motion while MdDS starts after the source of that motion has been removed, such as after disembarking a ship[47]. In fact, many MdDS patients indicate that their symptoms start immediately upon reaching dry land[41], while other patients state that their symptoms start the morning after a night of sleep[35].

Most often, patients experiencing MdDS report ongoing sensations of rocking (93% of patients) or swaying (81%) along with unsteadiness and disequilibrium when walking as well as when lying down long after the original source of these sensations (e.g.

boat, plane) has been removed[34]. As mentioned earlier, some of these symptoms can mimic what is reported with several other vestibular and neurological disorders. Because of this overlap, it is imperative that a proper diagnosis is obtained so as to provide the appropriate care.

In addition to the range of MdDS symptoms starting after passive-motion activities, some patients report symptoms occurring after amusement rides as well as in response to motion-type video games[48]. Others have attributed their symptoms to stress, changes in body position, or hormonal changes[27]. One study utilizing a survey to collect patient symptoms found incidents of disorientation, postural instability, imbalance, fatigue, impaired cognition, and kinesiophobia associated with MdDS[27]. In addition, to a lesser degree, patients have reported events such as nausea, jumping vision, headache, blurred vision, diplopia, vomiting, eye twitches, and other less common symptoms[49]. Unlike many other conditions that affect balance or equilibrium, however, the incidence of nausea, vomiting, or vertigo is quite rare with MdDS. Furthermore, MdDS does not appear to affect an individual's hearing[41].

While MdDS is known to exhibit symptoms that can also be found in other balance-related disorders, it also has a very unique characteristic not found in other conditions. For example, many MdDS patients report relief from their symptoms when they return to the type of passive motion that immediately preceded the start of their symptoms[29, 39]. In other words, returning to the boat or ship that caused their MdDS actually makes them feel better. Similarly, many patients report improvement when actively driving a car[41]. This characteristic is one of the key criteria used by some researchers for separating MdDS from other vestibular disorders[9]. Patients of other conditions such as phobic postural vertigo have been found to experience symptom relief when their condition is explained to them, but as with most dizziness-related disorders, re-exposure to the initial cause of their symptoms does not provide any relief[50].

While it's clear that the symptoms of MdDS are unique and often long-term, it is also important to point out that some patients do experience diminished symptoms after approximately six months[36]. Still, patients may experience the symptoms of MdDS for years or more, while a small portion report that their symptoms diminish but then later return[36]. Unfortunately, the longer symptoms are present, the less likelihood there will be for resolution of those symptoms[28].

Conclusion

There is no doubt that MdDS is a unique disease. Despite exhibiting symptoms that mimic many vestibular disorders, MdDS appears to be a relatively rare disease localized to the neural pathways within the central nervous system as compared to arising directly from within the vestibular organs of the ear. Despite this difference, MdDS does share some characteristics with certain vestibular disorders such as vestibular migraine or Meniere's disease in that it is more prevalent within an older as well as mostly female population. The range of symptoms associated with MdDS can vary significantly between patients yet does involve some degree of perceived motion that is often described as a rocking or swaying sensation. While other disorders capable of causing imbalance or unsteadiness may exhibit an improvement of symptoms in response to actions such as lying down, MdDS appears to be unaffected by any alterations in body position. Furthermore, returning a patient to the original source of motion that caused their MdDS (e.g. ship, airplane) typically causes short-term alleviation of the rocking or swaying sensations inherent to MdDS. Clearly, MdDS brings a unique challenge to the small group of people who experience the often debilitating symptoms after cruises, air travel, or even video game activity. In the next chapter, we'll focus on how these characteristics of MdDS are used to help establish a diagnosis in affected patients.

Chapter 4 – Diagnosis

In order to establish the presence of any particular disease, there has to be a set of criteria that defines the signs, symptoms, or test results that the disease accompanies. For example, a heart attack should not be diagnosed by a patient having 'chest pain' alone. After all, a weight lifter attempting a new personal-best in the bench press may have several subsequent days of chest pain. However, chest pain along with several additional factors (e.g. elevated blood proteins, shortness of breath) can be useful measures that contribute towards diagnosis of a heart attack. With any disease, the collective signs, symptoms, and test results used to establish the presence or absence of a disease is known as that disease's *diagnostic criteria.* Medical professionals use established criteria for a particular disease against the existing signs and symptoms to determine the presence or absence of disease. Sometimes, making the diagnosis is quite easy as there is a physical presence of something like a virus that clearly warrants a diagnosis of the common cold. In other cases, migraine may or may not be present during spells of vertigo that can make diagnosis of vestibular migraine somewhat tricky.

Unfortunately, MdDS does not yet have an established and accepted set of diagnostic criteria. As such, it has been stated that a finding of MdDS is often reached through a diagnosis of exclusion[51], which is to say that MdDS is diagnosed when all other possibilities have been ruled out. Possible explanations as to why MdDS may not yet have established diagnostic criteria could be that it is considered a rare disease, or it may be that symptoms often resolve over time without much medical intervention. Or, it might simply be that there is not yet enough attention focused on MdDS to have enough data to define what makes a true MdDS patient versus someone who exhibits symptoms such as random dizziness.

The lack of established diagnostic criteria is probably at least partly to blame for the relative obscurity that MdDS maintains within the medical community[29]. Without a set of guidelines dictating the criteria needed to diagnose a patient with MdDS, medical professionals do not have a clear path towards a diagnosis. Instead, patients exhibiting a sensation of rocking or swaying may be classified as 'dizzy', thereafter being sent home with some anti-nausea medicine and a recommendation to return if symptoms are not better within one month.

Although diagnostic criteria have not yet been accepted, they have been *proposed*. This means that researchers have looked at the common and consistent symptoms of MdDS and made an attempt to establish guidelines that separate MdDS from all other medical conditions. Because these guidelines have not yet been implemented, they remain proposed guidelines as of current. Hopefully, a medical community, society, or profession will elect to enact these or at least some other set of conditions in order to formally recognize the diagnostic criteria for MdDS.

The proposed set of diagnostic criteria as outlined by researchers Saha and Fife are as follows[41]:

A. Onset of symptoms after exposure to passive motion (a), such as following travel on a boat/cruise ship or airplane
B. Main symptom is illusory rocking motion
C. Symptoms improve with re-exposure to passive motion, such as boat or car travel
D. Nausea is not a prominent symptom
E. Minimum 3-month duration of symptoms (b)
F. Not better accounted for by another International Classification of Headache Disorders-3 diagnosis or by another vestibular disorder (c)

a: Exposure to passive motion must last at least several hours and more likely will have lasted days.

b: A diagnosis of MdDS may still be made with symptoms lasting less than 3 months; however, for a   diagnosis   of   persistent MdDS symptoms must have lasted at least 3 months.

c: History and physical do not suggest another vestibular disorder, or another disorder was considered but ruled out with appropriate testing, or another disorder is present but as an independent condition with episodes that can be clearly differentiated.

As indicated by these proposed guidelines, diagnosis with true MdDS requires at least three months of symptoms. Therefore, a patient complaining of a rocking sensation over the past month should not be diagnosed with the *syndrome* form of MdDS but might rather be a candidate for *transient* MdDS. Though such intricacies might seem trivial, the ability to differentiate between two or more medical conditions is vital for allowing medical professionals to reach a proper diagnosis. Ironically, these same intricacies contribute to why diagnostic criteria are difficult to establish, as they must be unique from all other medical conditions and also agreed upon by the organization, society, or profession that developed them. For example, if a group of neurologists read the above guidelines, they may disagree that 3 months of symptoms is required for a diagnosis of MdDS. If so, they may lobby to have their particular field of medicine NOT support such guidelines and instead call for only one month of symptoms. It can almost seem political at times, but there is a very real reason for establishing clear diagnostic criteria for diseases such as MdDS as it helps prevent overlap with other diseases and also ensures that people who truly have MdDS are not excluded simply because they do not meet all of the established criteria.

It is of interest to point out that MdDS patients have a history of being misdiagnosed with a mental disorder (e.g. depression)[42]. This is not to say that MdDS is associated with patients who have a mental disorder; rather, it may be that patients with MdDS exhibit the signs and symptoms of a mental disorder due to extraneous circumstances such as a lack of understanding from others, overall impact of MdDS itself, and a general lack of treatment options[29]. These associated events highlight the importance of not only recognizing MdDS as a medical condition but also ensuring proper and effective treatment of the associated issues as well.

Conclusion

Given the recent attention that MdDS has received from the research community, the awareness of MdDS is certain to increase. This increased awareness should be expected to benefit patients as over time there will likely

71

be greater recognition of MdDS within the medical community along with improved treatment options. Perhaps most importantly, the eventual establishment of official diagnostic criteria will help identify MdDS and separate it from several other medical conditions that produce similar symptoms. Furthermore, as MdDS receives additional attention, it is hoped that the attention will spur even more interest which will hopefully contribute favorably to research that will eventually lead to a consistent cure for patients.

Chapter 5 – Treatment

It's sad to have to be blunt when trying to provide the best information possible for a medical condition, but MdS warrants such a case. Unfortunately, there are *currently* not any effective treatments to cure MdDS. As we'll discuss in this chapter, though, there are promising treatments under development. This lack of a cure is somewhat common amongst disorders affecting equilibrium. Some disorders, like BPPV, can in fact be cured relatively quickly for most patients while others such as Ménière's disease and vestibular migraine have treatments that are effective for some patients but not others. And still other relatively complex conditions such as PPPD or MdDS are just too new in the medical field to have the years of targeted research that can be used to outline effective treatments, thereby leaving patients with treatments based on case reports or anecdotal evidence.

To help you sort out the high degree of treatment options that you may come across, we are going to first spend a good part of this chapter talking about how the scientific process is used to develop effective treatments. This chapter is *not* intended to teach you how to become a scientist – rather, it is written with the intent of helping you be able to weed out the good information from the bad, much of which you'll find online via outlets such as social media. Given the misery that MdDS can bring – including reports that it has driven patients to suicide[45] – it can be easy as a patient to be taken advantage of or fall victim to scam treatments. Therefore, the first part of this chapter will be spent on helping you understand a bit more about what is known as the *empirical research* process that is often used to help establish the effectiveness of a treatment. In taking time to learn about this process, I think it will help you become more adept at sorting fact from fiction when it comes to MdDS-based claims, sales pitches, and so-called 'miracle cures'.

The scientific process

Science is all about observations. If a researcher designs an experiment, he or she has already predicted an outcome more commonly known as the *hypothesis*. By observing what happens during an experiment, his or her hypothesis will be supported or rejected. In some cases, hypotheses are relatively simple, such as *if I flip a coin, it will reveal 'heads' 50% of the time.* There is pretty much a one-in-two chance that the coin will show 'heads', as there are only two sides to the coin. Therefore, such a hypothesis is quite simple to prove, for if you drop the coin enough times, it's highly likely that heads or tails will occur approximately 50% of the time.

One thing about good science is that it is never permitted to simply *assume*. As a researcher you still have to test your hypothesis in order to see if you were indeed correct. After all, there may be some unknown, small factor that influences your experiment. What if, for example, someone handed you a pair of die that when rolled, came up as a "three" and "four" 84% of the time? Wouldn't that seem a little odd versus what you would predict? If so, your hypothesis of expecting completely random numbers over and over would be refuted. A little further investigation may reveal that the dice were secretly altered so as to come up as a total of "7". So even though you expected that a pair of dice would provide random pairs of numbers, you still have to test your prediction to ensure that there is not some unknown factor influencing the results.

As I mentioned, making predictions using coins or dice are quite simple examples. Things get much more complicated in terms of experiments and predictions when it comes to fields like medicine or psychology. If a researcher designs a drug with the intent for that drug to cure a specific condition, it is relatively simple in concept to design the drug molecule to fit and bind to a specific receptor in the body that should generate an action that the researcher intends. However, it is much more complicated to get that drug molecule to the area of the body it needs to be, or survive the digestive system, or stay in an active form long enough for it to bind to its receptor. In addition, researchers also have to be able to predict any side-effects or unwanted conditions that may result from that drug; otherwise, even if a drug performs its intended duty, too serious of side effects would ultimately prevent its use. Furthermore, they have to show that whatever positive and negative effects occur do in fact occur consistently across several individuals with that condition. It can be a frustrating and difficult process, but it is essential for establishing the 'truth' and the safety specific to a drug or medical treatment.

Unfortunately, establishing all of these factors takes both time and money. A researcher typically has to obtain a grant in order to pay for the facilities, staff, and equipment to design and test their treatment (i.e. drug, machine, etc.) for a specific condition. On top of that, the researcher has to get approval from a board of experts before they are even allowed to begin their experiment, an often drawn-out process that serves to ensure that what the researcher is proposing is both ethical and necessary. And if the process reveals legitimate results – sometimes only in a test tube – the researcher has to be able to show that their results can be replicated (i.e. repeated) across a wide variety of individuals of various backgrounds and health statuses, yet another drawn-out process. Once that occurs and there is a clear and safe benefit in using the drug or product, the researcher will most likely be able to start marketing his or her product. When done properly, this process can take years.

In light of the effort required to develop and test a potential treatment effectively, many individuals and companies have decided that it's much simpler to just forego all of the bureaucratic 'nonsense' and post some treatment online that they believe is effective. The problem in doing so is that there often lacks real evidence that the treatment actually works. And, the person selling the treatment often knows that the product has no proof – especially when there is a potential for financial gain in store for them if they can just convince enough people to buy the product. It is up to the consumer or patient to be able to determine whether any claims made by the seller are in fact true or just a sales gimmick.

Testing on subjects

To outline why it is important that treatments work across groups of people rather than just a single person, we need to look at what is commonly referred to as a *subject*, or an individual involved in experimental testing.

Humans are very similar but very different from each other. Stand two individuals of the same gender, height, and weight next to each other and you might say that they are very similar. But, if you investigate deeper into what you can't see, you might find that one is allergic to a substance, or has high blood pressure, or maybe has an autoimmune disorder. In other words, looking at their outward appearance tells you nothing about particular details that you can't see, such as an underlying medical condition. So, what may be beneficial or safe for one of them might not be the case for both. However, if a researcher can show that a treatment works for *many* – even though it may not work for 'everyone' – it can be cause for getting that treatment approved and on the market.

In medicine, when something applies to a single entity, such as a person, location, or event, it is referred to as a *case*. For example, a flu outbreak at a school after a student returns from a trip would be specific to that school, and is not particularly relevant to *all* schools. Therefore, that particular flu outbreak could be considered a case for that school. Similarly, if a patient is allergic to, say bacon, that would make his or her situation a case specific to him or her rather than an expected reaction for everyone, as the vast majority of people are not allergic to bacon. Medical treatments apply similarly – if something works for one single patient, it doesn't necessarily mean that it is an effective treatment. Likewise, if one person cannot use a treatment due to an allergy or some other situation, it does not mean that 'all' individuals should not use the treatment. But, if a treatment works for many people in a variety of situations (i.e. a "pool" of individuals), it is much more likely that the treatment truly works.

When it comes to MdDS treatments and 'cures', you will probably find unique options available online. Expect, however, that most of these treatments have not only failed to go through the experimental design process as described earlier, but you will also likely find little evidence of consistent effects. Product descriptions may highlight a testimonial or two, but the question you as the patient and consumer have to ask yourself is whether that testimonial is valid and whether that positive comment is worth you purchasing the product. After all, it's no secret that people can get paid to make positive comments about a product.

To outline how a useless product can seem to some consumers to be a miracle cure, we can use the classic example of an old phone scam that perfectly outlines how people can fall for false promises. Say you are a swindler and you are needing some cash. You call 40 people, 20 to whom you tout a new, 'hot' stock "A" and 20 to whom you tout stock "B". Stock "A" ends up doing poorly, so you never call back that group. But stock "B" does well, so you call back those people and say "see, I *told* you it would do well!". Knowing that your potential victims aren't quite sold on your service, you then tell half of those remaining people to buy stock "C", and half to buy stock "D". But only stock "D" ends up doing well. Therefore, you quickly call back the people you told about stock "D", bragging about your skills as a stock genius and asking if they are finally ready to invest. Given what appeared to be your two hot recommendations, many in the group hand over money to you to invest for them. What the people in that group don't know is that 30 of your 40 original phone calls went unreturned due to a lack of product performance. Unfortunately for them, they are quick to hand you their money to invest – after which you skip town, never to be seen again.

Internet-based MdDS treatment options can work similarly. Sure, a person can tout the effects of a treatment, but for how many patients did the treatment *not* work well for? If a $10 treatment works on 20 people but does not work on 80, is that a financial risk? Perhaps not, and depending on the potential harm (hopefully there is none) it may be worth trying if nothing else has worked for a patient. But, what if that rarely successful treatment is a series of steps that take a month to complete, costs $400, and has the same 20% success rate? You might be a bit hesitant to partake in such a treatment, and you certainly should be skeptical.

When skepticism arises, your next step should be to simply investigate the claims made. Who made the claim? If the company is touting their own product or performed their own research on their own manufactured product, red flags – a lot of them – should be raised. If the product was tested independently, such as by a third-party researcher who has no ties to the company, it can greatly improve the validity of the product claims. But putting a product through the testing phase costs money, and it is often much easier to just market the product to desperate people and convince them that it works. Maybe even pay some consumers to write the aforementioned favorable testimonial which will most likely make it onto the product manufacturer's website. As potential customers look through the website, a bunch of positive reviews makes it tempting to purchase the product. But, isn't that really what effective marketing is supposed to do – convince you to buy a product? As the price you are willing to pay increases, you as the consumer and patient have to carefully decide if the product is worth the risk. And having solid information about how the product was tested can play an important role in your decision.

True effects vs coincidence

Along the same lines of establishing whether a product works on a single patient or is effective across a range of patients, it is also important to evaluate the facts about the treatment's reported effects. For example, say a person goes to a rock concert full of loud, booming speakers, and later that night has a good bit of ringing in his ear. A friend gives him an oil to put in his ear, and when he wakes up, the ringing is greatly diminished. The second day after the rock concert, and after a little bit more oil was applied, the ringing disappeared. Does that mean that the oil fixed his tinnitus? Or could it be that he simply didn't have the true chronic-type tinnitus that many individuals suffer from, and therefore it went away on its own?

Given the circumstances, it's highly likely that the rock concert caused temporary tinnitus that resolved itself in a few hours. Therefore the oil had no real effect at all; rather, it was just pure coincidence that the application of the oil coincided with the natural reduction in tinnitus. But what do you think might happen when a few years later that same person runs into a colleague who is complaining of constant ringing in her ear for the past six weeks? There's little doubt that he'll end up touting the effects of the oil that he is certain stopped his own tinnitus. And given the long-term status of her tinnitus, she'll probably want to give it a try.

This scenario outlines the classic situation where a misinterpretation of effects leads to belief in a treatment that doesn't really work. Unfortunately, with chronic conditions such as MdDS that can create patients who are desperate for relief, there are individuals that capitalize on this desperation in order to sell treatments that have no realistic chance of working. I often see it myself online, and that is the main reason for my adding this 'introduction to research' to the chapter – to make you as a patient and consumer more aware. So, let's look a little deeper into what you should be assessing when it comes to MdDS treatments.

Designing experiments

When science looks for a new treatment, it applies the treatment to one group (the experimental group) and no treatment to another identical group (the control group). Then, differences are evaluated between the groups, with the experimental group typically expected to have a favorable outcome. For example, if there was a belief that low iron intake caused MdDS, it could be *tested* by designing an appropriate experiment. The two groups would be equally comprised of individuals of similar gender and age as well as both duration and severity of MdDS. In other words, you wouldn't want to apply the new treatment to a group of, say, females, and then use all males in the control group. Rather, you want consistency in the makeup of the subjects between the two groups. Therefore, you would establish each group so that they consist of similar individuals (e.g. comparable MdDS duration, gender, age, etc.). Then, for the experiment you would add the iron supplements to a meal for the experimental group while supplying the same meal to the control group, but without the added iron supplement. As long as everything else stays the same, any consistent results occurring in the experimental group (such as an improvement in the majority of the group's MdDS symptoms after consuming the additional iron) should be expected to be due to the treatment, and not random coincidence. If there is no improvement in the experimental group after the additional iron intake, it could be determined that the treatment of iron supplementation has no effect.

We discussed how the makeup of the experiment and control group is important. If, as mentioned, the groups are not made of similar individuals, you would effectively be comparing apples to oranges and therefore, any results you obtain from the experiment would have no real validity. Besides physical makeup such as age and gender, similarity in symptoms between groups is important as well. For example, if you had one group that reported having mild sea sickness for six months and another group had debilitating MdDS for at least ten years, keeping them separated into individual experimental and control groups would result in a major study design flaw. However, if you *mixed* the groups so that some people with short-term and others with long-term symptoms and severity were in the same group, that would be acceptable as it creates a "pool' of subjects of similar conditions between the experimental and control groups.

It is also strongly recommended that the groups are comprised of enough people to capture the possible variations in the condition (i.e. MdDS) that could affect the results. Do the groups capture all severities of MdDS, or just a specific one or two types? Is the long-term group all taking a certain medication? Have they had a certain medical procedure? If so, these particular situations become *confounders* if they can influence the experiment's results. Say, for example, that ¾ of the people in the aforementioned experimental group were also taking an 'anti-nausea supplement' that interfered with iron absorption. If those same people then took the iron supplement, the iron would have no chance to exert its potential effects on MdDS. Therefore, the experiment's results may end up showing that only some of the people in the experimental group had an improvement in their MdDS symptoms after taking an iron supplement. If those same people were also the ones that were *not* taking the anti-nausea supplement, it would make the experiment's results look as though the iron was not very effective when in fact the iron was being prevented from working in the experimental group because some participants were taking the anti-nausea supplement. Therefore, study design is vital and must include aspects such as ensuring that the group's subjects are properly selected and screened, and confounding factors (such as some subjects taking a certain headache supplement) are controlled.

This may seem like a lot of detail for a MdDS patient to be worried about, but truth be told, these concepts should be a key factor in whether that consumer elects to try out a particular treatment. Truth be told, most medications have already gone through this process and should leave you little worry as to how they were developed. The bigger issue specific to effectiveness lies with supplements and – perhaps more importantly – online claims. If an individual or company is not willing to discuss how they arrived at their marketing claims such as *"reduced sensation of 'rocking' severity by 50%"*, it should immediately raise questions for anyone considering the treatment. For example, questions should be raised such as "Reduced in what population?" "How long was the treatment given?" "Did they have any other treatments or do anything else simultaneously?" "How and when was the rocking severity measured?" The more questions that can be answered legitimately, the more credibility the product gains. Do not be afraid to challenge any claim or product before you spend money on it!

There are certainly times when a treatment may only be tested and shown successful on a particular type of MdDS patient such as females, or only when patients have had sensations of tilting or rocking for less than a month, and that limited evidence is perfectly acceptable if the product is marketed as such. In those cases, it is fine to report the findings as long as the success is also reported to be *limited* to that particular population. Remember – assuming is not permitted when it comes to 'assuming' that a treatment reported in one group will apply similarly to another. In other words, if a treatment has not been tested on a particular type of MdDS patient, it cannot be assumed that the treatment will work until that factor is addressed using a reputable scientific study. So, if a treatment is shown to reduce the incidence of vertigo attacks in postmenopausal MdDS patients, it cannot be assumed that the product will also work equally well in males until that has been shown with a proper experiment.

What is all of this saying? Simple – it is recommended that you strive to look for treatments that have gone through the rigor of scientific testing if you're going to spend money on the treatment. There is actually much, much more that we could discuss regarding the scientific process and how it applies to MdDS treatment, as we have just skimmed the surface. But, what we have discussed should help you to ask questions and read with more detail the evidence behind treatments that you encounter.

If there is no clear evidence or indication of a treatment's proof, I strongly suggest that you look elsewhere. You can certainly try the product, but know that there are risks to your health as well as your wallet that should be addressed first. At the same time, I am cognizant that there is no cure yet for MdDS and as such, the cure remains 'out there' somewhere. As we continue to eliminate ineffective treatments, we strengthen the pool of effective options while also expanding our search into promising new areas. When considering an alternative treatment for your own MdDS, consider the financial cost, the physical risk including side effects, and the evidence that exists for the treatment. The degree of proof that is required in order to use a particular treatment is ultimately left up to you.

Summarizing the scientific process

You may have been wondering if we were ever going to get to the part about treatments for MdDS. The answer is certainly 'yes', but I wanted to include the previous material because it is important to me as an author that you understand how to wade through the vast amount of information that you will be presented with specific to treatment of MdDS. As a former researcher, I am immediately skeptical of any claim presented as anecdotal (i.e. personal experience) rather than based in the scientific process; that is just the effect of my years of research-based training and it is not exactly right or wrong as a belief. To a MdDS sufferer, though, living with the invasiveness of the constant perception of motion may lead them to try *anything* regardless of the purported benefits. And in many cases this can be ok as long as it doesn't cause physical or financial harm to you. But it can also lead to wasted time and false hope if you're not careful, and false hope often leads to repeated bouts of disappointment and/or depression as yet another hopeful cure falls flat. So, take the information you learned in this first part of the chapter and always be sure to perform your own level of evaluation of a treatment's effectiveness. If you happen to find something that works for you, by all means use it! It certainly doesn't *have* to have gone through the research process, particularly if it's a natural product (e.g. spice, herb). But if you are actively looking for treatments and read a claim online, look for the sources or research used to establish that claim. If you are told of a treatment that can help, ask what it is about the product that works, as well as how it works better than other available options. Being diligent about these claims can help ensure that you are making valuable progress toward a beneficial treatment that can help reduce your own symptoms.

Treatment Awareness for MdDS

As I said at the start of this chapter, there is not yet a cure for MdDS. That is to say only that there is currently no *cure* for MdDS – not that there is nothing out there that can provide patients some relief. Part of the reason for a lack of cure may lie in the fact that MdDS is just simply a disease that has only recently gained a directed research focus. As such, the timeframe for quality research to produce effective results just hasn't elapsed (remember from earlier in this chapter how we discussed the length of time it can take for true empirical research to become known!). As of yet, there are relatively few studies in existence that utilize control and experimental groups to study a particular treatment specifically for MdDS. Hopefully that will change as time progresses and we see more research growth towards MdDS.

Evaluating treatments – particularly for a relatively 'new' medical condition such as MdDS – requires extra diligence on the part of the patient as to the true effectiveness of those treatments. As we stated earlier in this chapter, it is possible that a medical condition (e.g. back pain) disappears on its own as a patient tries a new treatment. In such a case it's not the treatment that is making the difference; rather, it's the normal time course of injury healing that caused the improvement. Internet groups are rife with anecdotal treatment success stories, and while some claims are likely correct that there was indeed improvement in a patient's condition that timed well with a particular treatment, the question must be answered as to whether the condition improved *because* of a treatment. In other words, when conducting your own online research for MdDS treatments it is important that you take time to ask questions that have viable answers. To put it another way, seek a mix of *caveat emptor* (let the buyer beware) along with the old Russian proverb *trust, but verify*.

One final discussion related to treatment of balance-related disorders must be addressed. As we have discussed, MdDS is often not a singular condition itself but may instead be mixed in with issues such as depression, anxiety, or even another vestibular condition. In such cases, it is important for the patient and his or her medical professional to recognize whether the treatment is improving the imbalance disorder itself or if the treatment is affecting some other aspect. For example, if a patient with MdDS is having ongoing nervousness about being in social situations, he or she may elect to use cannabis due to its purported medical benefits. In a discussion with other MdDS sufferers, that patient may say something along the lines of "cannabis worked wonders for my MdDS". While such a claim is likely true, the question arises as to whether the cannabis helped the actual MdDS or whether it affected an ancillary effect of

MdDS such as anxiety. Cannabis is well-known for its anti-anxiety benefits, so a patient taking cannabis may, for example, feel less nervous about going out in public. Therefore, while cannabis was said to 'work wonders' for one patient's MdDS, a patient without anxiety may feel motivated to try it for his or her own MdDS only to find that is has no real benefit. The issue was not that cannabis didn't work, it was that the patient was experiencing its benefits for something *other* than actual MdDS.

For some patients, their MdDS disappears on its own after a period of time. In fact, minimizing the effects of MdDS while awaiting spontaneous resolution of symptoms is a recommended treatment strategy[36]. However, as we noted in an earlier chapter, the longer a patient has symptoms of MdDS, the less likely that the condition will resolve on its own[28]. The ability to rely on time itself as a treatment is largely a decision that should be made between the patient and his or her medical professional. Depending on the severity of the patient's symptoms, they may elect to pursue a more aggressive, less conservative option instead.

Medication has been shown to have mixed effects in treating MdDS. Drugs used to combat dizziness or motion sickness do not have any effect on active MdDS[41]. Benzodiazepines, which have anti-anxiety effects, have been shown to help alleviate symptoms for some MdDS patients, as have selective serotonin re-uptake inhibitors (SSRIs) that are known to have positive effects on combating depression[28]. Among smaller groups of 6-10 patients, clonazepam, diazepam, and alprazolam helped some but not all patients[49]. In fact, one survey-based study reported that benzodiazepines and antidepressant drugs provided the most effective symptom relief for their MdDS, so much so that the study authors recommended these drugs as a treatment for MdDS along with physical therapy[42]. Several other drugs that target symptoms such as motion sickness and dizziness along with those drugs that work as diuretics have not had much success in treating MdDS[28].

Dietary changes such as reduced sodium intake, which are known to have success in providing symptom relief for other vestibular conditions such as Ménière's disease[28], have also had no real effect at reducing the effects of MdDS.

Vestibular therapy (VT) is a type of therapy that aims to improve factors such as balance, dizziness, and unsteadiness. As a treatment, VT has several different types of therapy that can be applied. Habituation, for example, attempts to reduce a patient's symptoms by repeatedly exposing them to the original cause of the symptoms. MdDS is unique from other vestibular symptoms in that many patients do feel relief *during* the time that they are exposed to the original cause of their MdDS (e.g. on board a ship), yet the effects return immediately afterwards with little improvement. Therefore, habituation-based VT seems to provide relief for MdDS during treatment, but does not seem to improve the overall condition. Separately, there has been small but noticeable improvement in MdDS symptoms reported when using certain types of VT[28]; however, improvement is not consistent, as other studies have reported less favorable effects from VT[49]. More importantly, VT has not been shown successful in alleviating the actual perceived motions that MdDS patients commonly experience[45].

One of the more successful non-drug treatments shown to reduce the symptoms of MdDS focuses on the VOR that we discussed back in Chapter 1. This treatment, known as VOR modulation, assumes that the VOR does not function efficiently in MdDS patients[43]. When exposed to this treatment, which consists of the MdDS patient turning his or her head side-to-side at the same frequency as their perceived rocking, all while observing a moving image, patients reported a decrease in their symptoms. Furthermore, many patients noted that their symptoms disappeared after the treatment, while others claimed that their symptoms had diminished significantly even after four months.

In more complex treatment attempts, repeated transcranial magnetic stimulation (rTMS) has been studied to investigate its effects on the symptoms of MdDS. Traditionally, rTMS has been used for the treatment of depression and anxiety, but researchers proposed that it could have beneficial effects in the treatment of MdDS[52]. Results are relatively promising and have shown to reduce the oscillations experienced by patients of MdDS[53], but more testing is needed to know the true effectiveness as well as the long-term benefits. These findings do require further investigation, as one author contends that the underlying cause of MdDS lies within what is known as the velocity-storage portion of the brain – an area deep within the skull devoted to processing movements such as rotation – which due to its location may limit the effectiveness of magnetic stimulation[1].

Treatment of MdDS-related effects

While direct treatment of MdDS as a medical condition is and should be the primary goal of any therapy plan, it is also important to pay attention to the numerous ancillary factors that may accompany MdDS. These factors are particularly important given that there is not a quick fix for MdDS which in turn means that treatment will likely be ongoing. Such ancillary factors have been listed to include work-related issues, depression, or the unfortunate occurrence of suicidal tendencies that have been shown to be associated with MdDS[45]. Whereas not all of these issues are medical-related, patients dealing with the effects of MdDS may also benefit from professionals who work in the areas of social work or psychology as part of the overall treatment plan.

Conclusion

In a perfect world, the goal of any therapy plan would be to achieve complete relief from a medical condition. Certainly, many conditions are curable through the use of drug therapy or a well-designed rehabilitation program. Other conditions or diseases simply heal on their own. In the case of balance and/or equilibrium-related conditions, many fail to resolve on their own yet can be improved with targeted therapy. Unfortunately, MdDS is among the newest balance-related condition, and without decades of targeted research focused on MdDS there is not yet a roadmap that leads to a simple cure. Because MdDS treatments vary widely in terms of what works and what doesn't, patients must be in constant communication with their medical providers in order to provide viable feedback about the effectiveness of any recommended treatment. And, patients as well as medical providers should be open to exploring alternative treatments for MdDS while still being mindful of evaluating the legitimacy of unproven therapies.

Chapter 6 – Quality of Life

When it comes to being a patient, having a particular disease is only one part of the equation. How that disease affects you as a patient as well as those around you is a whole other aspect that must be accounted for and may even play a role in when and what type of treatment you select. The degree to which an individual is affected by his or her particular disease is outlined by what is known as *quality of life*. If, for example, a disease does not impact a patient's own standards for health, comfort, or happiness in their life, that disease is said to have no real impact on quality of life. On the other hand, if a disease limits a patient's social interaction, or causes pain throughout the day, or prevents them from doing things like making their own breakfast, that disease likely has a significant impact on the respective patient's quality of life.

No matter the degree of injury or illness, the effect that a disease can have on quality of life is largely dependent upon a patient's own perception of that disease. For example, a retiree afflicted with a constant sensation of 'rocking' may report a much higher quality of life than a single mom trying to support her child by working two jobs all while experiencing a similar degree of rocking-type sensation. Even if their degree of disability is the same, the impact that the sensations can have is likely higher for the single mom, thereby causing her to have a lower perceived quality of life. Simply put, few will argue that living with MdDS can have a profound impact on an individual's quality of life, and the research we'll discuss shortly serves to confirm as much.

Assessing quality of life

Given how personal perception can play a role in a patient's quality of life, it can be somewhat challenging to assess how an illness such as MdDS impacts daily life for a patient. Traditionally, quality of life is measured using patient surveys that have been tested and validated for accuracy. Unfortunately, given the variation between patients that can occur with MdDS (e.g. symptoms, treatment type, etc.), it can be difficult to gather enough data to form an effective evaluation that can outline quality of life in response to specific treatments. Furthermore, if a very generic survey is used to collect information, as often occurs in vestibular-based research, the resulting data may not be specific enough to clarify how a particular disease impacts the patient. For example, the Short-Form 36 (SF-36) survey asks 36 questions related to overall quality of life measures, and is commonly used as an assessment across a variety of health conditions. While well-accepted within the research and medical community, the SF-36 is not specific to MdDS. However, certain parts of the survey could be considered relevant to what MdDS patients deal with on a daily basis such as the impact of MdDS on the patient's ability to work or enjoy social functions[54].

Recently, MdDS-specific surveys were developed in order to collect information regarding patient characteristics as well as experiences with MdDS[42]. In developing a survey for MdDS patients, specific information can be collected that provides relevant information for researchers and will likely be useful in the future as well.

Patient vs. Physician Outcomes

As we discussed in the previous chapter, one of the main goals in the modern-day treatment of MdDS is not necessarily to eliminate the symptoms as much as make the patient comfortable until the symptoms abate on their own[36]. From a quality of life viewpoint, it would not be unexpected to find that most patients would rather accept a slight bit of tilting or rocking sensation as compared to undergoing more aggressive treatments that may have unwanted or permanent side effects. The resulting psychological, physical, and even financial consequences of treatment are all important aspects to consider when assessing quality of life specific to MdDS.

Until just the past 20 years or so, many treatment strategies have focused on what is known as physician-centered outcomes – those factors that medical professionals are typically interested in such as the degree of influence on a patient's gait pattern. In recent decades, however, treatment decisions have had much more patient input specific to what the patient feels is important such as recovery time, driving ability, or future quality of life issues. In separating physician-centered outcomes from those that are patient-centered, it helps point out that what a physician might see as effective treatment may not always match the patient's expectations simply because the anticipated outcomes are different[55]. For example, a physician may elect to simply monitor the patient to see if MdDS symptoms decrease over time despite the fact that the patient may feel that the impact of those symptoms on their ability to work necessitates more aggressive options. Ultimately, you the patient should be at the forefront of decisions made that are specific to your care, but those decisions should incorporate a balance of the most beneficial treatment mixed with the least impact on your daily life.

Quality of life with MdDS

We talked in an earlier chapter that MdDS patients report visiting up to 19 medical providers before receiving a diagnosis[40]. As such, the journey involved with MdDS can contribute quite a bit of stress to a patient's life. This stress likely contributes to why MdDS patients exhibit high levels of depression as well as anxiety. These psychological factors – in addition to stress itself – has been linked to both having a medical condition that is not well understood or recognized in medicine along with the overall 'intrusiveness' of the condition itself[44, 48]. It is important to highlight that the psychological issues associated with MdDS are not a cause for the condition but rather the effects of the condition[42]. In other words, a patient with MdDS who exhibits a high degree of anxiety is manifesting the effects of MdDS as anxiety – they should not be incorrectly classified as developing MdDS because they are anxious.

The stress involved in MdDS can be highlighted by reports indicating that if diagnosed with MdDS at a point in which the patient had 20 years of employment remaining, the economic impact for that patient would exceed $250,000! Along these same lines, almost a third of patients have reported that they sought a change in their employment due to MdDS[49].

MdDS has been shown to negatively affect quality of life. In fact, the range of quality of life scores in one particular study were on level with long-term multiple sclerosis[40]. Those MdDS patients reported low scores in physical and mental health, thereby exposing those personal areas deemed most affected by patients. More specifically, role limitations due to physical problems, energy, and emotional problems were singled out as having low quality of life scores. In contrast, pain and sexual function were reported to have the highest scores.

In the context of quality of life, intrusiveness relates to how much of an impact a particular illness has on certain aspects of life. Patients afflicted by MdDS were found to have significant intrusiveness, even more than scores reported for rheumatoid arthritis or end-stage renal disease. Researchers also reported that stigma scores of MdDS, which reflect the degree to which people feel judged by their medical condition, exceeded scores of epilepsy as well as episodic (but not chronic) migraine[48].

Conclusion

The research makes it clear that MdDS can negatively impact a patient's quality of life. For some, it may just be a matter of 'surviving the darkness' until their symptoms alleviate on their own. Others, however, may not experience relief from their MdDS symptoms, and those are the patients that are going to be in most need of effective intervention. Social and economic factors are shown to have negative effects on quality of life, and it is important that medical professionals consider interventions that can help minimize the impact of MdDS on a patient's life. In addition, patients must also be aware of the negative influence that MdDS can have and make the effort to instill positive changes during the time that they are exhibiting symptoms of MdDS. As quality of life improves, patient outcomes can be expected to improve as well. This in turn can help stave off potential negative consequence of MdDS such as depression or unnecessary stress that can cause further unnecessary burden to a patient.

Chapter 7 – A day in the life

To understand the constant aggravation and interruption that MdDS can bring, you have to be able to put yourself into the shoes of someone who actually lives with the condition. In many of my vestibular books I will set aside a chapter to outline what my own life can be like when impacted by my vestibular disorders. I feel that it not only highlights what can often be the misery that comes with a vestibular disorder, but it also serves to let other patients know that they are not alone as they can read first-hand what other sufferers must deal with. Whereas I only have to deal with transient MdD of an hour or so after a boat ride, I sought out someone who suffers from true MdDS and was willing to share their story. Next, you will read what a day in the life of MdDS is like for Lindsay, who has given me permission to share her story as follows.

'I did too much yesterday' I think as I force myself out of bed. The rocking started before I'd even opened my eyes. It's 9am - I slept twelve hours, the fatigue is still overwhelming. Maybe I got too stressed at my part time job, maybe I watched too much TV, perhaps it was the loud train I'd had to stop for...it is hard to tell most days. I run into the counter as I take the dogs outside...that's going to bruise. I take a breath and keep going. I feel like I'm walking on a trampoline - I used to think those were fun. As I stand outside waiting for my pups I find myself rocking side to side physically to try and match what I feel is happening - this is a technique I use to stave off nausea, I find myself doing it almost unconsciously now. I sit to re-evaluate my tasks for the day...I'd written them out yesterday in hopes today would be a less rocky day. Now I feel the all too familiar pang of guilt for only being able to accomplish the bare minimum again. Laundry, Dishes, Groceries. I'm moving much slower than on a good day. I make it through a few loads of laundry before the rocking kicks up from the up and down of loading and unloading the machines. In between loads I rest, I focus on my breathing, I repeat to myself that I am not my illness. I decide to order groceries for delivery. I'd rather be in charge of my own shopping, but the store can sometimes make the rocking worse...I'm not sure if it's the lighting or the crowd, but I've had some near floor experiences on my bad days that I'd like to avoid today. I make lunch...something easy that requires no prep. I start the dishes and nearly drop a water glass on the floor...I'm too clumsy for this today, my husband will finish them later. He will also make

106

dinner because I can't trust my hands enough to chop or cook, and he will most likely stay up long past me even though I'm going to nap and I slept so long last night. I take a breath and keep going. Laundry, Groceries. The doorbell rings and I hit the kitchen door frame as I go through...another bruise. I put away the groceries and sleep for an hour. Laundry. I've managed to get the dogs in and out without injuring myself again. I've also got the last load going and have officially counted this day as a win. I try to work on my website and art but the brain fog is intense today and I just can't concentrate. I relax till my husband comes home, we watch some TV, eat the food he's made. I call it a night at 8pm because my brain is screaming at me that it needs a break from this wonky-ness, lights and noises. In my dreams I don't usually rock.

I have more days like this than I'd like to admit. I'm 31 years old and five years into my MdDS adventure. I also suffer from Endometriosis which may contribute slightly to some of my bad days. Most days are better, my rocking is minimal and I can do so much more, keeping in mind that I still avoid triggers like rollercoasters, theatres and stress. Rarely do I have worse days, where I can't even get past the 'get out of bed' part - usually those happen after I travel. It is hard to get over how drastically my life has changed because of MdDS. Once I was diagnosed (2 years after onset) I started learning how to manage my symptoms - but so far managing is all I can do, and still I have days like this. I have called out of work and cancelled many plans with friends - they all know that my 'brain cloud' is not something I'm willing to test anymore. I'm thankful that my husband is here to help me, to make sure I don't fall down the stairs or chop off a finger. I count myself lucky to have support, lucky to not have to work a full-time job, and lucky I had some amazing life experiences before MdDS.

Chapter 8 – Related Conditions

Vestibular-related symptoms come in many shapes and sizes and are all capable of causing significant disability for the patient. The symptoms associated with MdDS often resemble those found with other inner-ear conditions, and as such it is of interest to note the *differences* that can exist between the many vestibular conditions which can cause symptoms such as unsteadiness, tinnitus, or hearing loss. Therefore, this chapter is designed to outline some of the more common medical conditions that can mimic the signs and symptoms associated with MdDS. In doing so, it not only highlights the similarities with MdDS but also outlines some key differences that can help medical professionals isolate MdDS as a potential culprit behind a patient's symptoms.

Ménière's disease

Ménière's disease is an illness thought to result from problems with the fluid regulation system of the inner ear. Ménière's patients typically experience an ongoing degree of unsteadiness and ear pressure or fullness intermixed with bouts of acute vertigo, nausea, and vomiting that can last several hours or more. Due in large part to the complexity and sensitivity of the vestibular system, Ménière's remains a complicated disease. While the acute vertigo attacks of Ménière's can be extremely debilitating, those attacks can be followed by months or years of almost no symptoms.

Several theorized causes of Ménière's have been proposed, including body water regulation issues, endolymph reabsorption anomalies, vascular abnormalities, and autoimmune factors. Of these possible causes, fluid regulation in the middle ear is considered to be one of the main triggers of Ménière's[56]. For example, water channels, which regulate the transport of water across membranes, have been implicated as a possible main cause of Ménière's[57]. This theory results from the idea that unexpected reductions or increases in the number of water channels can influence the balance of fluid on each side of a membrane, and any alteration in fluid balance can have negative consequences in the equilibrium system of the ear.

Similarly, some researchers suggest that Ménière's patients have a diminished capacity to regulate fluid within their inner ear[58]. Consequently, fluctuations in the inner ear fluid are not well tolerated in Ménière's patients. This is thought to lead to fluid imbalances that contribute to many of the symptoms encountered by Ménière's patients. Electrolytes such as sodium that are known to play a role in the body's fluid regulation are commonly restricted in Ménière's patients in order to reduce potential fluctuations within the middle ear.

Other theorized causes of Ménière's disease include autoimmune disorders[59], the herpes virus[60], cervical (i.e. neck) disorders[61] and stress[62]. Whereas no definitive cause of Ménière's has been discovered, it is vital that research continues to investigate these and all logical possibilities to determine the potential link and/or similarities between Ménière's and balance-related disorders such as MdDS. At present there remains no cure for Ménière's, though symptoms can often be controlled through the aforementioned sodium restriction, medication, intratympanic steroid injection, and if necessary, surgical procedures on the middle ear.

Benign paroxysmal positional vertigo

As we have discussed, one of the most common vertigo conditions seen in primary care is benign paroxysmal positional vertigo (BPPV)[63]. Despite the long name, each word plays a role in describing what occurs with the disease. Most patients with this relatively harmless (benign) condition describe sudden (i.e. paroxysmal) bouts of vertigo that occur with certain positional-dependent head positions.

The mechanism involved in BPPV is thought to be due to the presence of loose crystals (i.e. otoliths) within the semicircular canals of the ear. As otoliths are not normally present within the semicircular canals, certain head movements cause the loose otoliths to contact the delicate hair cells of the semicircular canals, causing them to trigger and falsely indicate body motion when the head is in particular positions. For example, patients with BPPV often report short bouts of vertigo when looking upwards or rolling over in bed[64]. Furthermore, nausea and vomiting can occur with more severe cases such as *intractable BPPV.*

Diagnosis of BPPV typically involves a thorough medical history and evaluation along with manipulating the head in an attempt to reproduce the symptoms. Most commonly, the Dix-Hallpike maneuver is used to attempt to reproduce the symptoms of BPPV. For this procedure, the patient is seated on a table and their head position is manipulated while the patient is put through a series of specific body positions. Because the otoliths will typically induce nystagmus along with vertigo, the patient's eyes are observed for nystagmus along with any patient-reported vertigo. Results of the Dix-Hallpike test are relatively reliable, being able to correctly identify patients with BPPV 83% of the time while correctly excluding patients without BPPV 52% of the time[63].

For those patients testing positive for BPPV, vestibular rehabilitation as well as canalith repositioning (e.g. Epley maneuver) are relatively successful. Vestibular rehabilitation typically consists of a series of head and/or body motions which may involve fixation of the eye on a single point. Pharmaceutical treatments are not recommended for use in the treatment of BPPV as research has shown no benefit[65]. It is also possible that BBPV symptoms return.

Vestibular migraine

Vestibular migraines are among the more common vestibular disorders, affecting up to 1% of the population[47, 66] and up to 11% of patients seeking treatment in dizziness-related clinics[67]. Vestibular migraines are also relatively common in children, having been reported to occur in nearly 3% of children aged 6-12 years of age[68]. Like Ménière's disease, vestibular migraine has no universally accepted definition, which can in turn limit recognition of vestibular migraines in affected patients. Only recently were the diagnostic criteria established which include the following[67].

1. Vestibular migraine

A. At least 5 episodes with vestibular symptoms of moderate or severe intensity, lasting 5 minutes to 72 hours

B. Current or previous history of migraine with or without aura according to the   International Classification of Headache Disorders (ICHD)

C. One or more migraine features with at least 50% of the vestibular episodes:

– headache with at least two of the following characteristics: one sided location, pulsating quality, moderate or severe pain intensity, aggravation by routine physical activity

– photophobia and phonophobia

– visual aura

D. Not better accounted for by another vestibular or ICHD diagnosis

2. Probable vestibular migraine

A. At least 5 episodes with vestibular symptoms of moderate or severe intensity, lasting 5 min to 72 hours

B. Only one of the criteria B and C for vestibular migraine is fulfilled (migraine history or migraine features during the episode)

C. Not better accounted for by another vestibular or ICHD diagnosis

The predominant symptoms of vestibular migraine include vertigo in combination with headache, and these two symptoms often occur relatively close to each other[64]. Other symptoms can include transient hearing fluctuations[69], nausea, vomiting, and a sensitivity to motion sickness[67]. Some patients have reported triggering of their migraine in response to dehydration, lack of sleep, or certain foods, but the relationship between these characteristics and vestibular migraines has not been well-studied[67]. Evidence of effective treatment of vestibular migraines is limited. Patients who respond favorably to anti-migraine medication have occurred, but the evidence is lacking as to overall effectiveness[70].

Persistent Postural-Perceptual Dizziness (PPPD)

As one of the most recently recognized vestibular disorders, our understanding of PPPD is quite limited. At present, no studies have determined the incidence or prevalence of PPPD, though the average patient is reported to be in their mid-40s, with a slightly higher occurrence rate in women[71]. Symptoms of PPPD are subjective in nature and do not exhibit any outward signs, but often include dizziness and/or unsteadiness that can fluctuate in severity[71]. These symptoms are often worsened when the patient has an upright posture[72] and are typically reduced when the patient lies down[71]. Movement, whether active or passive in nature, typically worsens the patient's symptoms, and the speed of the motion tends to correlate to the degree of symptoms that the patient experiences[71]. Patients also note that visual stimuli, such as shadows aligning a roadway or walking down a grocery store aisle can often exacerbate symptoms.

The cause of PPPD remains unknown, but given the relative 'newness' of PPPD as a medical condition, there will likely be an increase in the amount of research directed toward it. Most patients exhibit the symptoms of PPPD after a particular vestibular event such as BPPV or vestibular neuritis[73], though a vestibular event is not required, as stress or anxiety[73] or even head trauma can trigger the effects of PPPD[74]. This prior vestibular event may cause some degree of difficulty in allowing the brain to separate out the multiple balance and proprioception inputs which in turn leads to chronic dizziness[75].

Though no cure for PPPD exists at present, several treatment options have been shown effective for reducing symptoms. Vestibular rehabilitation[76], cognitive behavioral therapy[77], medication[78], and nerve stimulation have all shown promise at treating the symptoms of PPPD[79].

Vestibular neuritis

Vestibular neuritis is associated with vertigo, nausea, vomiting, and imbalance, and is thought to be due to viral inflammation of the vestibular nerve[80]. The condition is considered to be acute as symptoms typically last from a few days to several weeks, but up to half of patients suffering from vestibular neuritis can experience symptoms for a much longer time[81]. Vestibular neuritis has been reported to account for nearly 10% of all dizziness-related medical visits[82]. Interestingly, viral epidemics trigger an increased incidence of vestibular neuritis, lending evidence to its likely inflammatory origins[83].

Patients exhibiting vestibular neuritis will present with acute, severe vertigo[64]. The most severe attacks can last for one to two days and then gradually subside over the following weeks. Motion may worsen the vertigo, and some patients experience nausea and vomiting in conjunction with the vertigo[64]. Additional symptoms often include nystagmus along with a walking pattern in which the patient tends to lean toward the affected ear's side.

Treatment of vestibular neuritis includes symptomatic care along with vestibular rehabilitation, which can begin as soon as tolerable after cessation of immediate symptoms[64]. Vestibular rehabilitation has been reported to be successful when compared against no therapy[84]. If vestibular neuritis is severe, short-term hospitalization may be required[64].

Concussion

Even a hit to the head has the potential to cause significant balance or instability-related symptoms, and many of these symptoms mimic what one would expect from MdDS. Concussion is a type of traumatic brain injury that most often results from a direct hit to the head or a type of injury (e.g. whiplash) that causes the brain to move rapidly within the skull. Concussions are not uncommon, with over 3 million concussions thought to occur per year in the United States[85]. The cause of concussion can vary by age, as children and older adults most commonly experience concussion as a result of falls, while in adults the most common cause is motor vehicle accidents[86]. Athletic participation, especially high-contact sports such as football, hockey, or boxing is also a common cause for concussion and even includes a separate classification as *sport-related concussion*.

Like many vestibular-related symptoms, imaging through x-ray, MRI, CT scan, etc. is relatively ineffective at diagnosing concussion. Therefore, diagnosis is typically reliant upon the patient's history, description of the event that caused the concussion, and their symptoms. The range of symptoms that can occur in response to concussion can vary but do have a close resemblance to many of the symptoms of MdDS. Typically, symptoms of concussion are classified into three areas – cognitive, emotional, and psychological. Cognitive symptoms include difficulty concentrating or thinking (i.e. 'brain fog') in addition to difficulty with information retention. Emotional symptoms of concussion can include irritability, sadness, or general nervousness. Physical symptoms probably have the most similarity to MdDS as they can include balance issues, 'brain fog', difficulty concentrating, among others[86].

Treatment of concussion is generally successful at relieving the associated symptoms. One of the first lines of treatment for concussion is rest. This includes both cognitive rest such as avoiding or reducing tasks that require a significant amount of 'thinking' (e.g. homework, computer use, etc.) as well as physical rest that avoids strenuous activity. Avoidance of associated triggers such as bright lights and loud noise is also recommended[87].

One of the positive aspects of concussion is that, unlike many other vestibular conditions, proper treatment generally results in a full recovery. Some individuals do have extended symptoms (e.g. 3 or more months), but the majority of individuals who suffer a concussion have relief of symptoms in a week or less and are typically allowed to resume activity. Having a

119

concussion can predispose an individual to having a future concussion, so care must be taken to limit the opportunity for future concussions to occur.

Conclusion

With that, you have reached the end of what I hope has been an informative and beneficial book for you. Living with MdDS can be difficult enough, but when you don't understand what is going on with the disease you can end up with additional stress and frustration. As I mentioned in the introduction for this book, my goal in taking on the task of writing this book was to provide you with factual information that you can use to have meaningful conversations with your physician. Having made it through chapters outlining what MdDS is as well as its suspected causes, I hope that you feel more empowered about your condition and are able to begin to understand the complexity of the disease.

Given that MdDS is new on the list of recognized medical conditions, there is not a clear set of diagnostic or treatment guidelines established. Consequently, MdDS remains relatively unknown by many treating practitioners, leaving patients to either elect to pursue additional care or adopt a 'wait and see' approach to determine whether their symptoms improve over time. Unlike other treatable disorders that produce similar unsteadiness or imbalance symptoms such as BPPV, the complexity of MdDS as a medical condition – particularly the fact that its cause has not been determined – makes treatment difficult as there is no particular tissue or structure at which to direct treatment towards. However, given the rise in attention given to MdDS over the past twenty or so years, it is much more likely that researchers will be able to hone in on a cause and inevitably find effective treatment options for patients. Still, even those treatments that have shown promise have only been able to be tested on a small number of patients, meaning that true, experiment-based findings outlining the effectiveness of particular treatments still elude us.

This is not to say that we don't know anything about MdDS as a medical condition though, either. Clearly, it predominantly affects middle-aged women, appears to be localized within the neural pathways of the brain that influence balance, and does not appear to be related to – nor respond to medication affecting – motion sickness. While these aren't definitive causes, every tidbit of information helps researchers narrow down potential causes which in turn allows researchers to focus their efforts on fewer and fewer likely sources of MdDS. And the fewer potential disease causes hat remain, the more likely the culprit will be found.

Despite no current cure, the need for focused research must continue for this debilitating disease. As outlined in a prior chapter, people are still eager to take cruises as well as ride in boats and fly on planes, indicating that the incidence of MdDS will likely continue on for many years until a cure is found. Ultimately, one would hope that we eventually become able to prevent MdDS so that vacationers and individuals employed on boats can enjoy their vacations or complete their job assignment without incident. Until then, we have to remain hopeful for effective treatments that can adequately alleviate the symptoms associated with MdDS. While we are not there yet, we are getting closer to finding the cause and ultimately an effective treatment for MdDS. Given the surge in research over the past two decades, one has to hope that we are close to finding viable answers.

I hope that this book has provided some valuable information for you to use in your own MdDS research, and allows you to have focused and engaged conversations with your medical provider that can bring you the answers that you need. In the meantime, I wish you all the best in your continued journey with MdDS.

Resources for MdDS Patients

Mal de Debarquement Syndrome Foundation
    mddsfoundation.org

Vestibular Disorders Association
    https://vestibular.org/mal-de-debarquement

National Organization for Rare Disorders
    https://rarediseases.org/rare-diseases/mal-de-debarquement/

Google Scholar
    search "Mal de Debarquement"

References

1.   Dai, M., et al., *Treatment of the Mal de Debarquement syndrome: a 1-year follow-up.* Frontiers in neurology, 2017. **8**: p. 175.
2.   Ekdale, E.G., *Form and function of the mammalian inner ear.* Journal of anatomy, 2016. **228**(2): p. 324-337.
3.   Schuknecht, H. and R. Ruby, *Cupulolithiasis*, in *Otophysiology.* 1973, Karger Publishers. p. 434-443.
4.   Cha, Y.-H., Y.Y. Cui, and R.W. Baloh, *Comprehensive clinical profile of Mal de debarquement syndrome.* Frontiers in neurology, 2018. **9**.
5.   Bisdorff, A., et al., *Classification of vestibular symptoms: towards an international classification of vestibular disorders.* Journal of Vestibular Research, 2009. **19**(1, 2): p. 1-13.
6.   Lawal, O. and D. Navaratnam, *Causes of Central Vertigo*, in *Diagnosis and Treatment of Vestibular Disorders.* 2019, Springer. p. 363-375.
7.   Peng, B., *Cervical vertigo: historical reviews and advances.* World neurosurgery, 2018. **109**: p. 347-350.
8.   Lee, A., *Diagnosing the cause of vertigo: a practical approach.* Hong Kong Med J, 2012. **18**(4): p. 327-32.
9.   Dai, M., et al., *Readaptation of the vestibulo-ocular reflex relieves the mal de debarquement syndrome.* Frontiers in neurology, 2014. **5**: p. 124.
10.   Glover, J.C., *Vestibular System*, in *Encyclopedia of Neuroscience*, L.R. Squire, Editor. 2004, Academic Press: Oxford. p. 127-132.
11.   Florence, C.S., et al., *Medical costs of fatal and nonfatal falls in older adults.* Journal of the American Geriatrics Society, 2018. **66**(4): p. 693-698.
12.   Whitman, G.T., *Dizziness.* The American journal of medicine, 2018. **131**(12): p. 1431-1437.
13.   Muncie, H.L., S.M. Sirmans, and E. James, *Dizziness: Approach to Evaluation and Management.* American family physician, 2017. **95**(3): p. 154-162.

14. Neuhauser, H., et al., *Epidemiology of vestibular vertigo: a neurotologic survey of the general population.* Neurology, 2005. **65**(6): p. 898-904.
15. Tusa, R.J., *Dizziness.* Medical Clinics of North America, 2009. **93**(2): p. 263-271.
16. Neuhauser, H., *The epidemiology of dizziness and vertigo,* in *Handbook of clinical neurology.* 2016, Elsevier. p. 67-82.
17. Zamergrad, M., et al., *Common causes of vertigo and dizziness in different age groups of patients.* Bionanoscience, 2017. **7**(2): p. 259-262.
18. Lin, H.W. and N. Bhattacharyya, *Impact of dizziness and obesity on the prevalence of falls and fall-related injuries.* The Laryngoscope, 2014. **124**(12): p. 2797-2801.
19. Neuhauser, H.K., et al., *Burden of dizziness and vertigo in the community.* Archives of internal medicine, 2008. **168**(19): p. 2118-2124.
20. Whalley, M.G. and D.A. Cane, *A cognitive-behavioral model of persistent postural-perceptual dizziness.* Cognitive and Behavioral Practice, 2017. **24**(1): p. 72-89.
21. Ziegler, M.G. and R.R. Barager, *Postural hypotension and syncope,* in *Cardiovascular Disease in the Elderly.* 1993, Springer. p. 211-230.
22. Agrawal, Y., *Dizziness Demographics and Population Health.* Dizziness and Vertigo Across the Lifespan, 2018: p. 1.
23. Kesser, B.W. and A.T. Gleason, *Multisensory Imbalance and Presbystasis,* in *Diagnosis and Treatment of Vestibular Disorders.* 2019, Springer. p. 331-352.
24. Koch, A., et al., *The neurophysiology and treatment of motion sickness.* Deutsches Ärzteblatt International, 2018. **115**(41): p. 687.
25. Zhang, L.L., et al., *Motion sickness: current knowledge and recent advance.* CNS neuroscience & therapeutics, 2016. **22**(1): p. 15-24.
26. Roscoe, J.A. and S.E. Matteson, *Acupressure and acustimulation bands for control of nausea: a brief review.* American journal of obstetrics and gynecology, 2002. **186**(5): p. S244-S247.

27. Van Ombergen, A., et al., *Mal de debarquement syndrome: a systematic review.* Journal of neurology, 2016. **263**(5): p. 843-854.

28. Cha, Y.-H., et al., *Clinical features and associated syndromes of mal de debarquement.* Journal of neurology, 2008. **255**(7): p. 1038.

29. Mucci, V., et al., *Mal de debarquement syndrome: a survey on subtypes, misdiagnoses, onset and associated psychological features.* Journal of neurology, 2018. **265**(3): p. 486-499.

30. Mucci, V., et al., *Perspective: stepping stones to unraveling the pathophysiology of Mal de Debarquement syndrome with neuroimaging.* Frontiers in neurology, 2018. **9**: p. 42.

31. Adams, F., *The genuine works of Hippocrates.* Vol. 17. 1849: Sydenham society.

32. Darwin, E., *Zoonomia, vol. I or, the laws of organic life.* 2007: Echo Library.

33. Irwin, J., *THE PATHOLOGY OF SEA-SICKNESS.* The Lancet, 1881. **118**(3039): p. 907-909.

34. Brown, J.J. and R.W. Baloh, *Persistent mal de debarquement syndrome: a motion-induced subjective disorder of balance.* American journal of otolaryngology, 1987. **8**(4): p. 219-222.

35. Cha, Y.-H., *Mal de debarquement syndrome: new insights.* Annals of the New York Academy of Sciences, 2015. **1343**(1): p. 63.

36. Hain, T.C. and M. Cherchi, *Mal de débarquement syndrome,* in *Handbook of clinical neurology.* 2016, Elsevier. p. 391-395.

37. Gleghorn, D., B.C. Doudican, and Y.-H. Cha, *Psychological Measures of Individuals with Mal de Debarquement Syndrome (P2. 156).* 2018, AAN Enterprises.

38. Cha, Y.-H., *Less common neuro-otologic disorders.* Continuum: Lifelong Learning in Neurology, 2012. **18**(5): p. 1142-1157.

39. Cha, Y.-H. *Mal de debarquement.* in *Seminars in neurology.* 2009. © Thieme Medical Publishers.

40. Macke, A., A. LePorte, and B.C. Clark, *Social, societal, and economic burden of mal de debarquement syndrome.* Journal of neurology, 2012. **259**(7): p. 1326-1330.

41. Saha, K.C. and T.D. Fife, *Mal de débarquement syndrome: review and proposed diagnostic criteria.* Neurology: Clinical Practice, 2015. **5**(3): p. 209-215.

42. Canceri, J.M., et al., *Examination of Current Treatments and Symptom Management Strategies Used by Patients With Mal De Debarquement Syndrome.* Frontiers in Neurology, 2018. **9**: p. 943.

43. Cha, Y.-H. and S. Chakrapani, *Voxel based morphometry alterations in Mal de debarquement syndrome.* PLoS One, 2015. **10**(8): p. e0135021.

44. Cha, Y.-H., et al., *Metabolic and functional connectivity changes in mal de debarquement syndrome.* PLoS One, 2012. **7**(11): p. e49560.

45. Cohen, B., S.B. Yakushin, and C. Cho, *Hypothesis: the vestibular and cerebellar basis of the Mal de Debarquement syndrome.* Frontiers in Neurology, 2018. **9**: p. 28.

46. Gordon, C., et al., *Clinical features of mal de debarquement: adaptation and habituation to sea conditions.* Journal of Vestibular Research, 1995. **5**(5): p. 363-369.

47. Cherchi, M. and T.C. Hain, *Migraine-associated vertigo.* Otolaryngologic Clinics of North America, 2011. **44**(2): p. 367-375.

48. Arroll, M.A., et al., *The relationship between symptom severity, stigma, illness intrusiveness and depression in Mal de Debarquement Syndrome.* Journal of health psychology, 2016. **21**(7): p. 1339-1350.

49. Hain, T.C., P.A. Hanna, and M.A. Rheinberger, *Mal de debarquement.* Archives of Otolaryngology–Head & Neck Surgery, 1999. **125**(6): p. 615-620.

50. Pollak, L., et al., *Phobic postural vertigo: a new proposed entity.* IMAJ-RAMAT GAN-, 2003. **5**(10): p. 720-723.

51. Teitelbaum, P., *Mal de debarquement syndrome: a case report.* Journal of travel medicine, 2002. **9**(1): p. 51-52.

52. Cha, Y.-H., Y. Cui, and R.W. Baloh, *Repetitive transcranial magnetic stimulation for mal de debarquement syndrome.* Otology & neurotology:

official publication of the American Otological Society, American Neurotology Society [and] European Academy of Otology and Neurotology, 2013. **34**(1): p. 175.

53. Cha, Y.-H., D. Gleghorn, and B. Doudican, *Occipital and Cerebellar Theta Burst Stimulation for Mal De Debarquement Syndrome.* Otology & Neurotology, 2019. **40**(9): p. e928-e937.

54. Instrument Ware Jr, J. and C. Sherbourne, *The MOS 36-item short-form health survey (SF-36): I. Conceptual framework and item selection.* Medical care, 1992. **30**(6): p. 473-483.

55. Carlson, M.L., et al., *Long-term quality of life in patients with vestibular schwannoma: an international multicenter cross-sectional study comparing microsurgery, stereotactic radiosurgery, observation, and nontumor controls.* Journal of neurosurgery, 2015. **122**(4): p. 833-842.

56. Minor, L.B., D.A. Schessel, and J.P. Carey, *Meniere's disease.* Current opinion in neurology, 2004. **17**(1): p. 9-16.

57. Ishiyama, G., I. Lopez, and A. Ishiyama, *Aquaporins and Meniere's disease.* Current Opinion in Otolaryngology & Head and Neck Surgery, 2006. **14**(5): p. 332-336.

58. Rauch, S.D., *Clinical Hints and Precipitating Factors in Patients Suffering from Meniere's Disease.* Otolaryngologic Clinics of North America, 2010. **43**(5): p. 1011-1017.

59. Kangasniemi, E. and E. Hietikko, *The theory of autoimmunity in Meniere's disease is lacking evidence.* Auris Nasus Larynx, 2018. **45**(3): p. 399-406.

60. Vrabec, J.T., *Herpes simplex virus and Meniere's Disease.* The Laryngoscope, 2003. **113**(9): p. 1431-1438.

61. Bjorne, A., A. Berven, and G. Agerberg, *Cervical Signs and Symptoms in Patients with Meniere's Disease: A Controlled Study.* CRANIO®, 1998. **16**(3): p. 194-202.

62. Söderman, A.C.H., et al., *Stress as a Trigger of Attacks in Menière's Disease. A Case-Crossover Study.* The Laryngoscope, 2004. **114**(10): p. 1843-1848.

63. Hanley, K., *Symptoms of vertigo in general practice: a prospective study of diagnosis.* Br J Gen Pract, 2002. **52**(483): p. 809-812.

64. Wipperman, J., *Dizziness and vertigo.* Primary Care: Clinics in Office Practice, 2014. **41**(1): p. 115-131.

65. Bhattacharyya, N., et al., *Clinical practice guideline: benign paroxysmal positional vertigo.* Otolaryngology--Head and Neck Surgery, 2008. **139**(5_suppl): p. 47-81.

66. Neuhauser, H., et al., *Migrainous vertigo Prevalence and impact on quality of life.* Neurology, 2006. **67**(6): p. 1028-1033.

67. Lempert, T., et al., *Vestibular migraine: diagnostic criteria.* Journal of Vestibular Research, 2012. **22**(4): p. 167-172.

68. Abu-Arafeh, I. and G. Russell, *Paroxysmal vertigo as a migraine equivalent in children: a population-based study.* Cephalalgia, 1995. **15**(1): p. 22-25.

69. Johnson, G.D., *Medical management of migraine-related dizziness and vertigo.* The Laryngoscope, 1998. **108**(S85): p. 1-28.

70. Fotuhi, M., et al., *Vestibular migraine: a critical review of treatment trials.* Journal of neurology, 2009. **256**(5): p. 711-716.

71. Staab, J.P., et al., *Diagnostic criteria for persistent postural-perceptual dizziness (PPPD): consensus document of the committee for the classification of vestibular disorders of the bárány society.* Journal of Vestibular Research, 2017. **27**(4): p. 191-208.

72. Staab, J.P., *Chronic subjective dizziness.* CONTINUUM: Lifelong Learning in Neurology, 2012. **18**(5): p. 1118-1141.

73. Trinidade, A. and J.A. Goebel, *Persistent Postural-Perceptual Dizziness—A Systematic Review of the Literature for the Balance Specialist.* Otology & Neurotology, 2018. **39**(10): p. 1291-1303.

74. Popkirov, S., J.P. Staab, and J. Stone, *Persistent postural-perceptual dizziness (PPPD): a common, characteristic and treatable cause of chronic dizziness.* Practical neurology, 2018. **18**(1): p. 5-13.

75. Lee, J.O., et al., *Altered brain function in persistent postural perceptual dizziness: A study on resting state*

132

functional connectivity. Human brain mapping, 2018. **39**(8): p. 3340-3353.

76. Staab, J.P., *Behavioral aspects of vestibular rehabilitation.* NeuroRehabilitation, 2011. **29**(2): p. 179-183.

77. Edelman, S., A.E. Mahoney, and P.D. Cremer, *Cognitive behavior therapy for chronic subjective dizziness: a randomized, controlled trial.* American journal of otolaryngology, 2012. **33**(4): p. 395-401.

78. Yu, Y.-C., et al., *Cognitive behavior therapy as augmentation for sertraline in treating patients with persistent postural-perceptual dizziness.* BioMed research international, 2018. **2018**.

79. Palm, U., et al., *Transcranial direct current stimulation (tDCS) for treatment of phobic postural vertigo: an open label pilot study.* European archives of psychiatry and clinical neuroscience, 2019. **269**(2): p. 269-272.

80. Schuknecht, H.F. and K. Kitamura, *Vestibular neuritis.* Annals of Otology, Rhinology & Laryngology, 1981. **90**(1_suppl): p. 1-19.

81. Perols, J.B., Olle, *Vestibular neuritis: a follow-up study.* Acta oto-laryngologica, 1999. **119**(8): p. 895-899.

82. Neuhauser, H.K. and T. Lempert. *Vertigo: epidemiologic aspects.* in *Seminars in neurology.* 2009. © Thieme Medical Publishers.

83. Baloh, R.W. and V. Honrubia, *Clinical neurophysiology of the vestibular system.* 2001: Oxford University Press, USA.

84. Hillier, S.L. and M. McDonnell, *Vestibular rehabilitation for unilateral peripheral vestibular dysfunction.* The Cochrane Library, 2011.

85. Brain Injury Research Institute. *What is a concussion?* ; Available from: http://www.protectthebrain.org/.

86. Centers for Disease Control and Prevention, *Traumatic Brain Injury and Concussion.* 2019.

87. Broglio, S.P., et al., *National Athletic Trainers' Association position statement: management of sport concussion.* Journal of athletic training, 2014. **49**(2): p. 245-265.

Let others know!

If you found this or any of Mark's other books informative, *please take the time and post a review online*! Reviews help get exposure for the books and thereby improve the chances that others will be able to benefit from the material as well.

Image Credits

Cover image: TAW4/shutterstock.com
Image 1.1: ilusmedical/shutterstock.com
Image 1.2: maxcreatnz/shutterstock.com
Image 1.3: designua/shutterstock.com
Image 1.4: designua/shutterstock.com

Check out these other books by Mark Knoblauch

Challenge the Hand You Were Dealt: Strategies to battle back against adversity and improve your chances for success

Essentials of Writing and Publishing Your Self-Help Book

Living Low Sodium: A guide for understanding our relationship with sodium and how to be successful in adhering to a low-sodium diet

Outlining Tinnitus: A comprehensive guide to help you break free of the ringing in your ears

Overcoming Ménière's: How changing your lifestyle can change your life

Professional Writing in Kinesiology and Sports Medicine

Seven Ways To Make Running Not Suck

The Art of Efficiency: A guide for improving task management in the home to help maximize your leisure time

Understanding BPPV: Outlining the causes and effects of Benign Paroxysmal Positional Vertigo

Vestibular Migraine: A Comprehensive Patient Guide

PPPD: A patient's guide to understanding persistent postural-perceptual dizziness

About the Author

Mark is a small-town Kansas native who now lives in a suburb of Houston with his wife and two young daughters. His background is in the area of sports medicine, obtaining his bachelor's degree from Wichita State and his master's degree from the University of Nevada, Las Vegas. After working clinically as an athletic trainer for eight years, Mark returned to graduate school where he received his doctorate in Kinesiology from the University of Houston, followed by a postdoctoral assistantship in Molecular Physiology and Biophysics at Baylor College of Medicine in Houston, TX. He has been employed as a college professor at the University of Houston since 2013

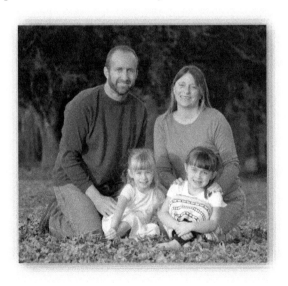